50% OFF CCM Certification Prep Course!

By Mometrix

Dear Customer,

We consider it an honor and a privilege that you chose our CCM Study Guide. As a way of showing our appreciation and to help us better serve you, we are offering **50% off our online CCM Prep Course.** Many CCM courses are needlessly expensive and don't deliver enough value. With our course, you get access to the best CCM prep material, and **you only pay half price**.

We have structured our online course to perfectly complement your printed study guide. The CCM Certification Prep Course contains **in-depth lessons** that cover all the most important topics, video reviews that explain difficult concepts, over **1,450+ practice questions** to ensure you feel prepared, and more than **350 flashcards** for studying on the go.

Online CCM Prep Course

Topics Include:

- Care Delivery and Reimbursement Methods
  - Models of Care
  - Continuum of Care
- Psychosocial Concepts and Support Systems
  - Behavioral Change Therapy
  - Wellness and Illness Prevention
- Quality and Outcomes Evaluation and Measurements
  - Data Interpretation and Reporting
  - Health Care Analytics
- Rehabilitation Concepts and Strategies
  - Adaptive Technologies
  - Vocational Aspects of Disabilities
- Ethical, Legal, and Practice Standards
  - Legal and Regulatory Requirements
  - Risk Management

Course Features:

- CCM Study Guide
  - Get content that complements our best-selling study guide.
- Full-Length Practice Tests
  - With over 1,450 practice questions, you can test yourself again and again.
- Mobile Friendly
  - If you need to study on the go, the course is easily accessible from your mobile device.
- CCM Flashcards
  - Our course includes a flashcard mode consisting of over 350 content cards to help you study.

To receive this discount, visit our website at mometrix.com/university/ccm or simply scan this QR code with your smartphone. At the checkout page, enter the discount code: **ccm50off**

If you have any questions or concerns, please contact us at support@mometrix.com.

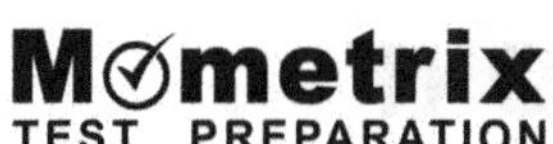

FREE Study Skills Videos/DVD Offer

Dear Customer,

Thank you for your purchase from Mometrix! We consider it an honor and a privilege that you have purchased our product and we want to ensure your satisfaction.

As part of our ongoing effort to meet the needs of test takers, we have developed a set of Study Skills Videos that we would like to give you for FREE. These videos cover our *best practices* for getting ready for your exam, from how to use our study materials to how to best prepare for the day of the test.

All that we ask is that you email us with feedback that would describe your experience so far with our product. Good, bad, or indifferent, we want to know what you think!

To get your FREE Study Skills Videos, you can use the **QR code** below, or send us an **email** at studyvideos@mometrix.com with *FREE VIDEOS* in the subject line and the following information in the body of the email:

- The name of the product you purchased.
- Your product rating on a scale of 1-5, with 5 being the highest rating.
- Your feedback. It can be long, short, or anything in between. We just want to know your impressions and experience so far with our product. (Good feedback might include how our study material met your needs and ways we might be able to make it even better. You could highlight features that you found helpful or features that you think we should add.)

If you have any questions or concerns, please don't hesitate to contact me directly.

Thanks again!

Sincerely,

Jay Willis
Vice President
jay.willis@mometrix.com
1-800-673-8175

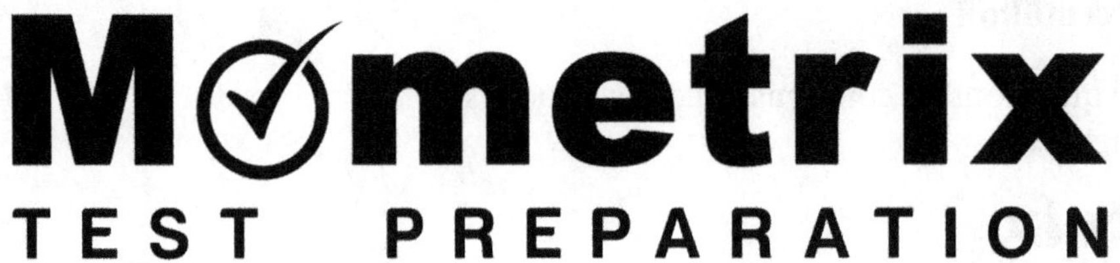

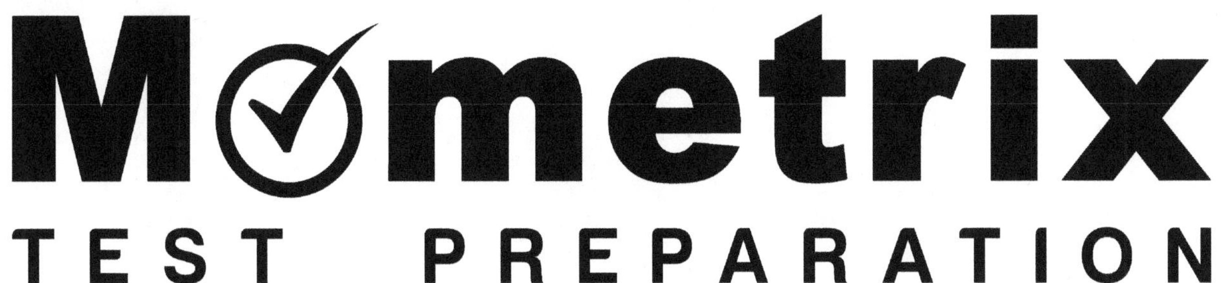

CCM

Certification Study Guide 2025-2026

600+ Practice Test Questions

Case Manager Exam Prep Secrets with Detailed Answer Explanations

7th Edition

Written and edited by Matthew Bowling

This paper meets the requirements of ANSI/NISO Z39.48-1992 (Permanence of Paper).

Paperback
ISBN 13: 978-1-5167-2727-8
ISBN 10: 1-5167-2727-4

DEAR FUTURE EXAM SUCCESS STORY

First of all, **THANK YOU** for purchasing Mometrix study materials!

Second, congratulations! You are one of the few determined test-takers who are committed to doing whatever it takes to excel on your exam. **You have come to the right place.** We developed these study materials with one goal in mind: to deliver you the information you need in a format that's concise and easy to use.

In addition to optimizing your guide for the content of the test, we've outlined our recommended steps for breaking down the preparation process into small, attainable goals so you can make sure you stay on track.

We've also analyzed the entire test-taking process, identifying the most common pitfalls and showing how you can overcome them and be ready for any curveball the test throws you.

Standardized testing is one of the biggest obstacles on your road to success, which only increases the importance of doing well in the high-pressure, high-stakes environment of test day. Your results on this test could have a significant impact on your future, and this guide provides the information and practical advice to help you achieve your full potential on test day.

Your success is our success

We would love to hear from you! If you would like to share the story of your exam success or if you have any questions or comments in regard to our products, please contact us at **800-673-8175** or **support@mometrix.com**.

Thanks again for your business and we wish you continued success!

Sincerely,
The Mometrix Test Preparation Team

Need more help? Check out our flashcards at:
http://mometrixflashcards.com/CCM

TABLE OF CONTENTS

Introduction

Thank you for purchasing this resource! You have made the choice to prepare yourself for a test that could have a huge impact on your future, and this guide is designed to help you be fully ready for test day. Obviously, it's important to have a solid understanding of the test material, but you also need to be prepared for the unique environment and stressors of the test, so that you can perform to the best of your abilities.

For this purpose, the first section that appears in this guide is the **Secret Keys**. We've devoted countless hours to meticulously researching what works and what doesn't, and we've boiled down our findings to the five most impactful steps you can take to improve your performance on the test. We start at the beginning with study planning and move through the preparation process, all the way to the testing strategies that will help you get the most out of what you know when you're finally sitting in front of the test.

We recommend that you start preparing for your test as far in advance as possible. However, if you've bought this guide as a last-minute study resource and only have a few days before your test, we recommend that you skip over the first two Secret Keys since they address a long-term study plan.

If you struggle with **test anxiety**, we strongly encourage you to check out our recommendations for how you can overcome it. Test anxiety is a formidable foe, but it can be beaten, and we want to make sure you have the tools you need to defeat it.

Secret Key #1 – Plan Big, Study Small

There's a lot riding on your performance. If you want to ace this test, you're going to need to keep your skills sharp and the material fresh in your mind. You need a plan that lets you review everything you need to know while still fitting in your schedule. We'll break this strategy down into three categories.

Information Organization

Start with the information you already have: the official test outline. From this, you can make a complete list of all the concepts you need to cover before the test. Organize these concepts into groups that can be studied together, and create a list of any related vocabulary you need to learn so you can brush up on any difficult terms. You'll want to keep this vocabulary list handy once you actually start studying since you may need to add to it along the way.

Time Management

Once you have your set of study concepts, decide how to spread them out over the time you have left before the test. Break your study plan into small, clear goals so you have a manageable task for each day and know exactly what you're doing. Then just focus on one small step at a time. When you manage your time this way, you don't need to spend hours at a time studying. Studying a small block of content for a short period each day helps you retain information better and avoid stressing over how much you have left to do. You can relax knowing that you have a plan to cover everything in time. In order for this strategy to be effective though, you have to start studying early and stick to your schedule. Avoid the exhaustion and futility that comes from last-minute cramming!

Study Environment

The environment you study in has a big impact on your learning. Studying in a coffee shop, while probably more enjoyable, is not likely to be as fruitful as studying in a quiet room. It's important to keep distractions to a minimum. You're only planning to study for a short block of time, so make the most of it. Don't pause to check your phone or get up to find a snack. It's also important to **avoid multitasking**. Research has consistently shown that multitasking will make your studying dramatically less effective. Your study area should also be comfortable and well-lit so you don't have the distraction of straining your eyes or sitting on an uncomfortable chair.

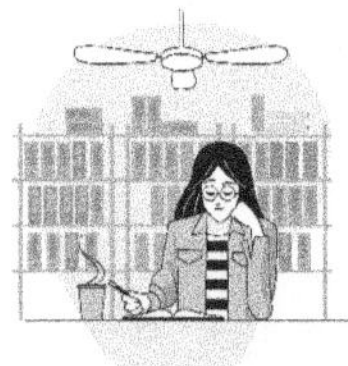

The time of day you study is also important. You want to be rested and alert. Don't wait until just before bedtime. Study when you'll be most likely to comprehend and remember. Even better, if you know what time of day your test will be, set that time aside for study. That way your brain will be used to working on that subject at that specific time and you'll have a better chance of recalling information.

Finally, it can be helpful to team up with others who are studying for the same test. Your actual studying should be done in as isolated an environment as possible, but the work of organizing the information and setting up the study plan can be divided up. In between study sessions, you can discuss with your teammates the concepts that you're all studying and quiz each other on the details. Just be sure that your teammates are as serious about the test as you are. If you find that your study time is being replaced with social time, you might need to find a new team.

Secret Key #2 – Make Your Studying Count

You're devoting a lot of time and effort to preparing for this test, so you want to be absolutely certain it will pay off. This means doing more than just reading the content and hoping you can remember it on test day. It's important to make every minute of study count. There are two main areas you can focus on to make your studying count.

Retention

It doesn't matter how much time you study if you can't remember the material. You need to make sure you are retaining the concepts. To check your retention of the information you're learning, try recalling it at later times with minimal prompting. Try carrying around flashcards and glance at one or two from time to time or ask a friend who's also studying for the test to quiz you.

To enhance your retention, look for ways to put the information into practice so that you can apply it rather than simply recalling it. If you're using the information in practical ways, it will be much easier to remember. Similarly, it helps to solidify a concept in your mind if you're not only reading it to yourself but also explaining it to someone else. Ask a friend to let you teach them about a concept you're a little shaky on (or speak aloud to an imaginary audience if necessary). As you try to summarize, define, give examples, and answer your friend's questions, you'll understand the concepts better and they will stay with you longer. Finally, step back for a big picture view and ask yourself how each piece of information fits with the whole subject. When you link the different concepts together and see them working together as a whole, it's easier to remember the individual components.

Finally, practice showing your work on any multi-step problems, even if you're just studying. Writing out each step you take to solve a problem will help solidify the process in your mind, and you'll be more likely to remember it during the test.

Modality

Modality simply refers to the means or method by which you study. Choosing a study modality that fits your own individual learning style is crucial. No two people learn best in exactly the same way, so it's important to know your strengths and use them to your advantage.

For example, if you learn best by visualization, focus on visualizing a concept in your mind and draw an image or a diagram. Try color-coding your notes, illustrating them, or creating symbols that will trigger your mind to recall a learned concept. If you learn best by hearing or discussing information, find a study partner who learns the same way or read aloud to yourself. Think about how to put the information in your own words. Imagine that you are giving a lecture on the topic and record yourself so you can listen to it later.

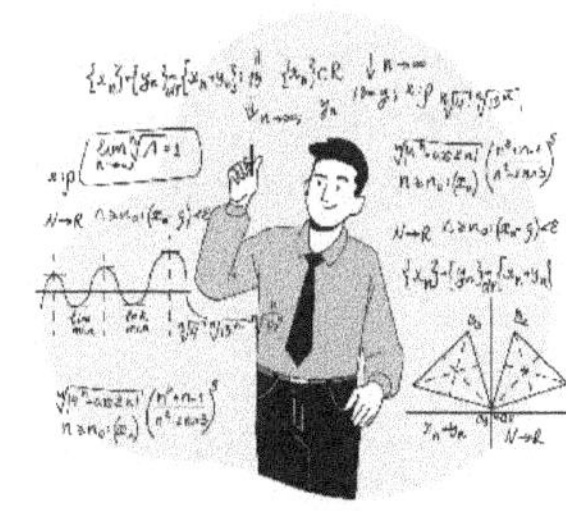

For any learning style, flashcards can be helpful. Organize the information so you can take advantage of spare moments to review. Underline key words or phrases. Use different colors for different categories. Mnemonic devices (such as creating a short list in which every item starts with the same letter) can also help with retention. Find what works best for you and use it to store the information in your mind most effectively and easily.

Secret Key #3 – Practice the Right Way

Your success on test day depends not only on how many hours you put into preparing, but also on whether you prepared the right way. It's good to check along the way to see if your studying is paying off. One of the most effective ways to do this is by taking practice tests to evaluate your progress. Practice tests are useful because they show exactly where you need to improve. Every time you take a practice test, pay special attention to these three groups of questions:

- The questions you got wrong
- The questions you had to guess on, even if you guessed right
- The questions you found difficult or slow to work through

This will show you exactly what your weak areas are, and where you need to devote more study time. Ask yourself why each of these questions gave you trouble. Was it because you didn't understand the material? Was it because you didn't remember the vocabulary? Do you need more repetitions on this type of question to build speed and confidence? Dig into those questions and figure out how you can strengthen your weak areas as you go back to review the material.

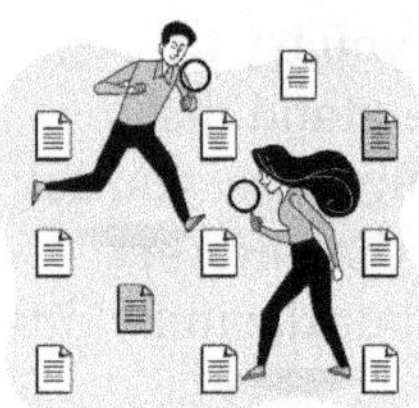

Additionally, many practice tests have a section explaining the answer choices. It can be tempting to read the explanation and think that you now have a good understanding of the concept. However, an explanation likely only covers part of the question's broader context. Even if the explanation makes perfect sense, **go back and investigate** every concept related to the question until you're positive you have a thorough understanding.

As you go along, keep in mind that the practice test is just that: practice. Memorizing these questions and answers will not be very helpful on the actual test because it is unlikely to have any of the same exact questions. If you only know the right answers to the sample questions, you won't be prepared for the real thing. **Study the concepts** until you understand them fully, and then you'll be able to answer any question that shows up on the test.

It's important to wait on the practice tests until you're ready. If you take a test on your first day of study, you may be overwhelmed by the amount of material covered and how much you need to learn. Work up to it gradually.

On test day, you'll need to be prepared for answering questions, managing your time, and using the test-taking strategies you've learned. It's a lot to balance, like a mental marathon that will have a big impact on your future. Like training for a marathon, you'll need to start slowly and work your way up. When test day arrives, you'll be ready.

Start with the strategies you've read in the first two Secret Keys—plan your course and study in the way that works best for you. If you have time, consider using multiple study resources to get different approaches to the same concepts. It can be helpful to see difficult concepts from more than one angle. Then find a good source for practice tests. Many times, the test website will suggest potential study resources or provide sample tests.

Practice Test Strategy

If you're able to find at least three practice tests, we recommend this strategy:

Untimed and Open-Book Practice

Take the first test with no time constraints and with your notes and study guide handy. Take your time and focus on applying the strategies you've learned.

Timed and Open-Book Practice

Take the second practice test open-book as well, but set a timer and practice pacing yourself to finish in time.

Timed and Closed-Book Practice

Take any other practice tests as if it were test day. Set a timer and put away your study materials. Sit at a table or desk in a quiet room, imagine yourself at the testing center, and answer questions as quickly and accurately as possible.

Keep repeating timed and closed-book tests on a regular basis until you run out of practice tests or it's time for the actual test. Your mind will be ready for the schedule and stress of test day, and you'll be able to focus on recalling the material you've learned.

Secret Key #4 – Pace Yourself

Once you're fully prepared for the material on the test, your biggest challenge on test day will be managing your time. Just knowing that the clock is ticking can make you panic even if you have plenty of time left. Work on pacing yourself so you can build confidence against the time constraints of the exam. Pacing is a difficult skill to master, especially in a high-pressure environment, so **practice is vital**.

Set time expectations for your pace based on how much time is available. For example, if a section has 60 questions and the time limit is 30 minutes, you know you have to average 30 seconds or less per question in order to answer them all. Although 30 seconds is the hard limit, set 25 seconds per question as your goal, so you reserve extra time to spend on harder questions. When you budget extra time for the harder questions, you no longer have any reason to stress when those questions take longer to answer.

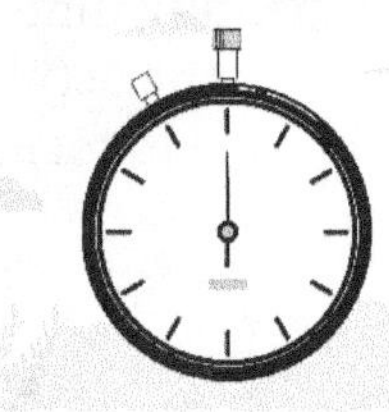

Don't let this time expectation distract you from working through the test at a calm, steady pace, but keep it in mind so you don't spend too much time on any one question. Recognize that taking extra time on one question you don't understand may keep you from answering two that you do understand later in the test. If your time limit for a question is up and you're still not sure of the answer, mark it and move on, and come back to it later if the time and the test format allow. If the testing format doesn't allow you to return to earlier questions, just make an educated guess; then put it out of your mind and move on.

On the easier questions, be careful not to rush. It may seem wise to hurry through them so you have more time for the challenging ones, but it's not worth missing one if you know the concept and just didn't take the time to read the question fully. Work efficiently but make sure you understand the question and have looked at all of the answer choices, since more than one may seem right at first.

Even if you're paying attention to the time, you may find yourself a little behind at some point. You should speed up to get back on track, but do so wisely. Don't panic; just take a few seconds less on each question until you're caught up. Don't guess without thinking, but do look through the answer choices and eliminate any you know are wrong. If you can get down to two choices, it is often worthwhile to guess from those. Once you've chosen an answer, move on and don't dwell on any that you skipped or had to hurry through. If a question was taking too long, chances are it was one of the harder ones, so you weren't as likely to get it right anyway.

On the other hand, if you find yourself getting ahead of schedule, it may be beneficial to slow down a little. The more quickly you work, the more likely you are to make a careless mistake that will affect your score. You've budgeted time for each question, so don't be afraid to spend that time. Practice an efficient but careful pace to get the most out of the time you have.

Secret Key #5 – Have a Plan for Guessing

When you're taking the test, you may find yourself stuck on a question. Some of the answer choices seem better than others, but you don't see the one answer choice that is obviously correct. What do you do?

The scenario described above is very common, yet most test takers have not effectively prepared for it. Developing and practicing a plan for guessing may be one of the single most effective uses of your time as you get ready for the exam.

In developing your plan for guessing, there are three questions to address:

- When should you start the guessing process?
- How should you narrow down the choices?
- Which answer should you choose?

When to Start the Guessing Process

Unless your plan for guessing is to select C every time (which, despite its merits, is not what we recommend), you need to leave yourself enough time to apply your answer elimination strategies. Since you have a limited amount of time for each question, that means that if you're going to give yourself the best shot at guessing correctly, you have to decide quickly whether or not you will guess.

Of course, the best-case scenario is that you don't have to guess at all, so first, see if you can answer the question based on your knowledge of the subject and basic reasoning skills. Focus on the key words in the question and try to jog your memory of related topics. Give yourself a chance to bring the knowledge to mind, but once you realize that you don't have (or you can't access) the knowledge you need to answer the question, it's time to start the guessing process.

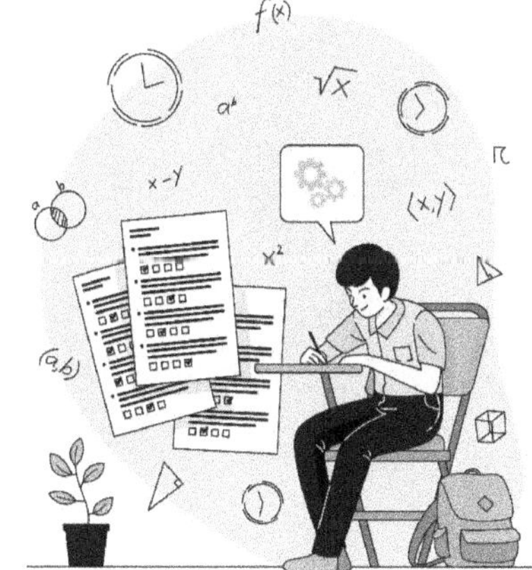

It's almost always better to start the guessing process too early than too late. It only takes a few seconds to remember something and answer the question from knowledge. Carefully eliminating wrong answer choices takes longer. Plus, going through the process of eliminating answer choices can actually help jog your memory.

Summary: Start the guessing process as soon as you decide that you can't answer the question based on your knowledge.

How to Narrow Down the Choices

The next chapter in this book (**Test-Taking Strategies**) includes a wide range of strategies for how to approach questions and how to look for answer choices to eliminate. You will definitely want to read those carefully, practice them, and figure out which ones work best for you. Here though, we're going to address a mindset rather than a particular strategy.

Your odds of guessing an answer correctly depend on how many options you are choosing from.

Number of options left	5	4	3	2	1
Odds of guessing correctly	20%	25%	33%	50%	100%

You can see from this chart just how valuable it is to be able to eliminate incorrect answers and make an educated guess, but there are two things that many test takers do that cause them to miss out on the benefits of guessing:

- Accidentally eliminating the correct answer
- Selecting an answer based on an impression

We'll look at the first one here, and the second one in the next section.

To avoid accidentally eliminating the correct answer, we recommend a thought exercise called **the $5 challenge**. In this challenge, you only eliminate an answer choice from contention if you are willing to bet $5 on it being wrong. Why $5? Five dollars is a small but not insignificant amount of money. It's an amount you could afford to lose but wouldn't want to throw away. And while losing $5 once might not hurt too much, doing it twenty times will set you back $100. In the same way, each small decision you make—eliminating a choice here, guessing on a question there—won't by itself impact your score very much, but when you put them all together, they can make a big difference. By holding each answer choice elimination decision to a higher standard, you can reduce the risk of accidentally eliminating the correct answer.

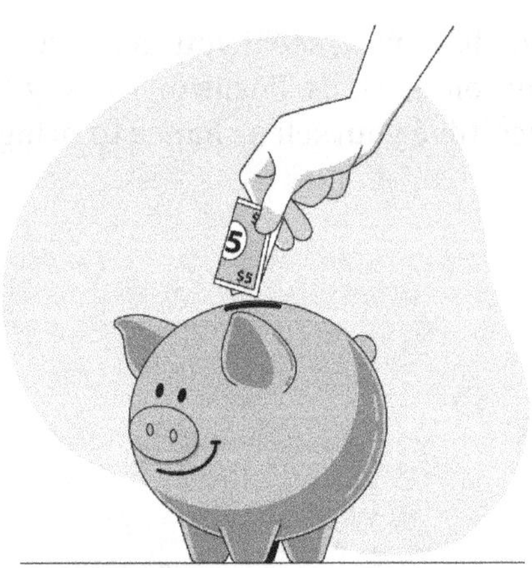

The $5 challenge can also be applied in a positive sense: If you are willing to bet $5 that an answer choice *is* correct, go ahead and mark it as correct.

Summary: Only eliminate an answer choice if you are willing to bet $5 that it is wrong.

Which Answer to Choose

You're taking the test. You've run into a hard question and decided you'll have to guess. You've eliminated all the answer choices you're willing to bet $5 on. Now you have to pick an answer. Why do we even need to talk about this? Why can't you just pick whichever one you feel like when the time comes?

The answer to these questions is that if you don't come into the test with a plan, you'll rely on your impression to select an answer choice, and if you do that, you risk falling into a trap. The test writers know that everyone who takes their test will be guessing on some of the questions, so they intentionally write wrong answer choices to seem plausible. You still have to pick an answer though, and if the wrong answer choices are designed to look right, how can you ever be sure that you're not falling for their trap? The best solution we've found to this dilemma is to take the decision out of your hands entirely. Here is the process we recommend:

Once you've eliminated any choices that you are confident (willing to bet $5) are wrong, select the first remaining choice as your answer.

Whether you choose to select the first remaining choice, the second, or the last, the important thing is that you use some preselected standard. Using this approach guarantees that you will not be enticed into selecting an answer choice that looks right, because you are not basing your decision on how the answer choices look.

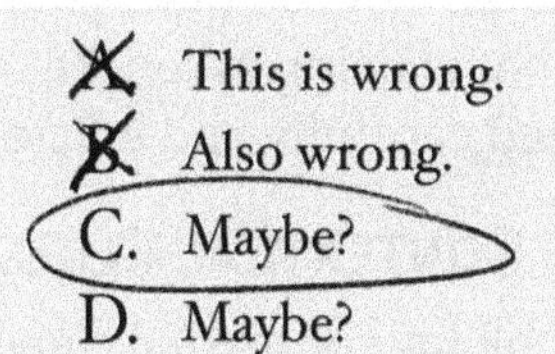

A. This is wrong.
B. Also wrong.
C. Maybe?
D. Maybe?

This is not meant to make you question your knowledge. Instead, it is to help you recognize the difference between your knowledge and your impressions. There's a huge difference between thinking an answer is right because of what you know, and thinking an answer is right because it looks or sounds like it should be right.

Summary: To ensure that your selection is appropriately random, make a predetermined selection from among all answer choices you have not eliminated.

Test-Taking Strategies

This section contains a list of test-taking strategies that you may find helpful as you work through the test. By taking what you know and applying logical thought, you can maximize your chances of answering any question correctly!

It is very important to realize that every question is different and every person is different: no single strategy will work on every question, and no single strategy will work for every person. That's why we've included all of them here, so you can try them out and determine which ones work best for different types of questions and which ones work best for you.

Question Strategies

READ CAREFULLY

Read the question and the answer choices carefully. Don't miss the question because you misread the terms. You have plenty of time to read each question thoroughly and make sure you understand what is being asked. Yet a happy medium must be attained, so don't waste too much time. You must read carefully and efficiently.

CONTEXTUAL CLUES

Look for contextual clues. If the question includes a word you are not familiar with, look at the immediate context for some indication of what the word might mean. Contextual clues can often give you all the information you need to decipher the meaning of an unfamiliar word. Even if you can't determine the meaning, you may be able to narrow down the possibilities enough to make a solid guess at the answer to the question.

PREFIXES

If you're having trouble with a word in the question or answer choices, try dissecting it. Take advantage of every clue that the word might include. Prefixes can be a huge help. Usually, they allow you to determine a basic meaning. *Pre-* means before, *post-* means after, *pro-* is positive, *de-* is negative. From prefixes, you can get an idea of the general meaning of the word and try to put it into context.

HEDGE WORDS

Watch out for critical hedge words, such as *likely, may, can, sometimes, often, almost, mostly, usually, generally, rarely,* and *sometimes.* Question writers insert these hedge phrases to cover every possibility. Often an answer choice will be wrong simply because it leaves no room for exception. Be on guard for answer choices that have definitive words such as *exactly* and *always.*

SWITCHBACK WORDS

Stay alert for *switchbacks.* These are the words and phrases frequently used to alert you to shifts in thought. The most common switchback words are *but, although,* and *however.* Others include *nevertheless, on the other hand, even though, while, in spite of, despite,* and *regardless of.* Switchback words are important to catch because they can change the direction of the question or an answer choice.

⊘ Face Value

When in doubt, use common sense. Accept the situation in the problem at face value. Don't read too much into it. These problems will not require you to make wild assumptions. If you have to go beyond creativity and warp time or space in order to have an answer choice fit the question, then you should move on and consider the other answer choices. These are normal problems rooted in reality. The applicable relationship or explanation may not be readily apparent, but it is there for you to figure out. Use your common sense to interpret anything that isn't clear.

Answer Choice Strategies

⊘ Answer Selection

The most thorough way to pick an answer choice is to identify and eliminate wrong answers until only one is left, then confirm it is the correct answer. Sometimes an answer choice may immediately seem right, but be careful. The test writers will usually put more than one reasonable answer choice on each question, so take a second to read all of them and make sure that the other choices are not equally obvious. As long as you have time left, it is better to read every answer choice than to pick the first one that looks right without checking the others.

⊘ Answer Choice Families

An answer choice family consists of two (in rare cases, three) answer choices that are very similar in construction and cannot all be true at the same time. If you see two answer choices that are direct opposites or parallels, one of them is usually the correct answer. For instance, if one answer choice says that quantity x increases and another either says that quantity x decreases (opposite) or says that quantity y increases (parallel), then those answer choices would fall into the same family. An answer choice that doesn't match the construction of the answer choice family is more likely to be incorrect. Most questions will not have answer choice families, but when they do appear, you should be prepared to recognize them.

⊘ Eliminate Answers

Eliminate answer choices as soon as you realize they are wrong, but make sure you consider all possibilities. If you are eliminating answer choices and realize that the last one you are left with is also wrong, don't panic. Start over and consider each choice again. There may be something you missed the first time that you will realize on the second pass.

⊘ Avoid Fact Traps

Don't be distracted by an answer choice that is factually true but doesn't answer the question. You are looking for the choice that answers the question. Stay focused on what the question is asking for so you don't accidentally pick an answer that is true but incorrect. Always go back to the question and make sure the answer choice you've selected actually answers the question and is not merely a true statement.

⊘ Extreme Statements

In general, you should avoid answers that put forth extreme actions as standard practice or proclaim controversial ideas as established fact. An answer choice that states the "process should be used in certain situations, if..." is much more likely to be correct than one that states the "process should be discontinued completely." The first is a calm rational statement and doesn't even make a definitive, uncompromising stance, using a hedge word *if* to provide wiggle room, whereas the second choice is far more extreme.

⊘ BENCHMARK

As you read through the answer choices and you come across one that seems to answer the question well, mentally select that answer choice. This is not your final answer, but it's the one that will help you evaluate the other answer choices. The one that you selected is your benchmark or standard for judging each of the other answer choices. Every other answer choice must be compared to your benchmark. That choice is correct until proven otherwise by another answer choice beating it. If you find a better answer, then that one becomes your new benchmark. Once you've decided that no other choice answers the question as well as your benchmark, you have your final answer.

⊘ PREDICT THE ANSWER

Before you even start looking at the answer choices, it is often best to try to predict the answer. When you come up with the answer on your own, it is easier to avoid distractions and traps because you will know exactly what to look for. The right answer choice is unlikely to be word-for-word what you came up with, but it should be a close match. Even if you are confident that you have the right answer, you should still take the time to read each option before moving on.

General Strategies

⊘ TOUGH QUESTIONS

If you are stumped on a problem or it appears too hard or too difficult, don't waste time. Move on! Remember though, if you can quickly check for obviously incorrect answer choices, your chances of guessing correctly are greatly improved. Before you completely give up, at least try to knock out a couple of possible answers. Eliminate what you can and then guess at the remaining answer choices before moving on.

⊘ CHECK YOUR WORK

Since you will probably not know every term listed and the answer to every question, it is important that you get credit for the ones that you do know. Don't miss any questions through careless mistakes. If at all possible, try to take a second to look back over your answer selection and make sure you've selected the correct answer choice and haven't made a costly careless mistake (such as marking an answer choice that you didn't mean to mark). This quick double check should more than pay for itself in caught mistakes for the time it costs.

⊘ PACE YOURSELF

It's easy to be overwhelmed when you're looking at a page full of questions; your mind is confused and full of random thoughts, and the clock is ticking down faster than you would like. Calm down and maintain the pace that you have set for yourself. Especially as you get down to the last few minutes of the test, don't let the small numbers on the clock make you panic. As long as you are on track by monitoring your pace, you are guaranteed to have time for each question.

⊘ DON'T RUSH

It is very easy to make errors when you are in a hurry. Maintaining a fast pace in answering questions is pointless if it makes you miss questions that you would have gotten right otherwise. Test writers like to include distracting information and wrong answers that seem right. Taking a little extra time to avoid careless mistakes can make all the difference in your test score. Find a pace that allows you to be confident in the answers that you select.

⊘ KEEP MOVING

Panicking will not help you pass the test, so do your best to stay calm and keep moving. Taking deep breaths and going through the answer elimination steps you practiced can help to break through a stress barrier and keep your pace.

Final Notes

The combination of a solid foundation of content knowledge and the confidence that comes from practicing your plan for applying that knowledge is the key to maximizing your performance on test day. As your foundation of content knowledge is built up and strengthened, you'll find that the strategies included in this chapter become more and more effective in helping you quickly sift through the distractions and traps of the test to isolate the correct answer.

Now that you're preparing to move forward into the test content chapters of this book, be sure to keep your goal in mind. As you read, think about how you will be able to apply this information on the test. If you've already seen sample questions for the test and you have an idea of the question format and style, try to come up with questions of your own that you can answer based on what you're reading. This will give you valuable practice applying your knowledge in the same ways you can expect to on test day.

Good luck and good studying!

Four-Week CCM Study Plan

On the next few pages, we've provided an optional study plan to help you use this study guide to its fullest potential over the course of four weeks. If you have eight weeks available and want to spread it out more, spend two weeks on each section of the plan.

Below is a quick summary of the subjects covered in each week of the plan.

- Week 1: Care Management & Reimbursement Methods
- Week 2: Psychosocial Concepts and Support Systems & Quality and Outcomes Evaluation and Measurements
- Week 3: Rehabilitation Concepts and Strategies & Ethical, Legal, and Practice Standards
- Week 4: Practice Tests

Please note that not all subjects will take the same amount of time to work through.

Three full-length practice tests are included in this study guide. We recommend saving the third practice test and any additional tests for after you've completed the study plan. Take these practice tests without any reference materials a day or two before the real thing as practice runs to get you in the mode of answering questions at a good pace.

Week 1: Care Management & Reimbursement Methods

Instructional Content

First, read carefully through the Care Management & Reimbursement Methods chapters in this book, checking off your progress as you go:

- ❑ Caseload Assignment and Selection
- ❑ Levels of Care and Care Settings
- ❑ Models of Care
- ❑ Lifespan Considerations
- ❑ Alternative Care Facilities
- ❑ Cost Containment and Financial Resources
- ❑ End-of-Life Care
- ❑ Interdisciplinary Care and Negotiation
- ❑ Management of Clients with Illness
- ❑ Physical Functioning and Behavioral Health Assessment
- ❑ Roles and Functions of Case Managers and Other Providers
- ❑ Continuum of Care
- ❑ Insurance Principles
- ❑ Reimbursement and Payment Methodologies
- ❑ Private Benefit Programs
- ❑ Public Benefit Programs
- ❑ Military Benefit Programs
- ❑ Utilization Management Principles
- ❑ Coding Methodologies
- ❑ Negotiation Techniques

As you read, do the following:

- Highlight any sections, terms, or concepts you think are important
- Draw an asterisk (*) next to any areas you are struggling with
- Watch the review videos to gain more understanding of a particular topic
- Take notes in your notebook or in the margins of this book

After you've read through everything, go back and review any sections that you highlighted or that you drew an asterisk next to, referencing your notes along the way.

Week 2: Psychosocial Concepts and Support Systems & Quality and Outcomes Evaluation and Measurements

Instructional Content

First, read carefully through the Psychosocial Concepts and Support Systems & Quality and Outcomes Evaluation and Measurements chapters in this book, checking off your progress as you go:

- ❑ Abuse and Neglect
- ❑ Behavioral Change Theory
- ❑ Behavioral Health Concepts and Systems
- ❑ Client Empowerment and Self-Care Management
- ❑ Community Resources
- ❑ Conflict Resolution and Crisis Intervention
- ❑ Interpersonal Communication
- ❑ Multicultural, Spiritual, and Religious Factors
- ❑ Neuropsychological Assessment
- ❑ Supportive Care Programs
- ❑ Wellness and Illness Prevention
- ❑ Data Interpretation and Reporting
- ❑ Health Care Analytics
- ❑ Quality and Performance Improvement
- ❑ Quality Indicators
- ❑ Evidence-Based Care Guidelines

As you read, do the following:

- Highlight any sections, terms, or concepts you think are important
- Draw an asterisk (*) next to any areas you are struggling with
- Take notes in your notebook or in the margins of this book

After you've read through everything, go back and review any sections that you highlighted or that you drew an asterisk next to, referencing your notes along the way.

Week 3: Rehabilitation Concepts and Strategies & Ethical, Legal, and Practice Standards

Instructional Content

First, read carefully through the Rehabilitation Concepts and Strategies & Ethical, Legal, and Practice Standards chapters in this book, checking off your progress as you go:

- ❑ Adaptive Technologies
- ❑ Vocational Aspects of Disabilities
- ❑ Vocational and Rehabilitation Delivery Systems
- ❑ Case Recording and Documentation
- ❑ Ethics Related to Care Delivery and Professional Practice
- ❑ Health Care and Disability Related Legislation
- ❑ Legal and Regulatory Requirements in Case Management
- ❑ Risk Management
- ❑ Case Manager Self-Care and Standards of Practice

As you read, do the following:

- Highlight any sections, terms, or concepts you think are important
- Draw an asterisk (*) next to any areas you are struggling with
- Watch the review videos to gain more understanding of a particular topic
- Take notes in your notebook or in the margins of this book

After you've read through everything, go back and review any sections that you highlighted or that you drew an asterisk next to, referencing your notes along the way.

Week 4: Practice Tests

Your success on test day depends not only on how many hours you put into preparing, but also on whether you prepared the right way. It's good to check along the way to see if your studying is paying off. One of the most effective ways to do this is by taking practice tests to evaluate your progress. Practice tests are useful because they show exactly where you need to improve. Every time you take a practice test, pay special attention to these three groups of questions:

- The questions you got wrong
- The questions you had to guess on, even if you guessed right
- The questions you found difficult or slow to work through

This will show you exactly what your weak areas are, and where you need to devote more study time. Ask yourself why each of these questions gave you trouble. Was it because you didn't understand the material? Was it because you didn't remember the vocabulary? Do you need more repetitions on this type of question to build speed and confidence? Dig into those questions and figure out how you can strengthen your weak areas as you go back to review the material.

Practice Test #1

Now that you've read over the instructional content, it's time to take a practice test. Complete Practice Test #1. Take this test with **no time constraints**, and feel free to reference the applicable sections of this guide as you go. Once you've finished, check your answers against the provided answer key. For any questions you answered incorrectly, review the answer rationale, and then **go back and review** the applicable sections of the book. The goal in this stage is to understand why you answered the question incorrectly, and make sure that the next time you see a similar question, you will get it right.

Practice Test #2

Next, complete Practice Test #2. This time, give yourself **3 hours** to complete all of the questions. You should again feel free to reference the guide and your notes, but be mindful of the clock. If you run out of time before you finish all of the questions, mark where you were when time expired, but go ahead and finish taking the practice test. Once you've finished, check your answers against the provided answer key, and as before, review the answer rationale for any that you answered incorrectly and then go back and review the associated instructional content. Your goal is still to increase understanding of the content but also to get used to the time constraints you will face on the test.

As you go along, keep in mind that the practice test is just that: practice. Memorizing these questions and answers will not be very helpful on the actual test because it is unlikely to have any of the same exact questions. If you only know the right answers to the sample questions, you won't be prepared for the real thing. **Study the concepts** until you understand them fully, and then you'll be able to answer any question that shows up on the test.

Care Management

Transform passive reading into active learning! After immersing yourself in this chapter, put your comprehension to the test by taking a quiz. The insights you gained will stay with you longer this way. Scan the QR code to go directly to the chapter quiz interface for this study guide. If you're using a computer, simply visit the bonus page at **mometrix.com/bonus948/ccm** and click the Chapter Quizzes link.

Caseload Assignment and Selection

Case Management

Definition

The Case Management Society of America defines case management as "a collaborative process of assessment, planning, facilitation, care coordination, evaluation, and advocacy for options and services to meet an individual's and family's comprehensive health needs through communication and available resources to promote patient safety, quality of care, and cost-effective outcomes."

Philosophy

Case management is fundamentally based on the tenet that **everyone benefits** when a client achieves optimal wellness and functional capacity: the client, the client's support system, the healthcare system, and those responsible for the cost of the client's care. Case management is a means to achieve these ends of client wellness and autonomy.

Values

Case management is a **collaborative** and **transdisciplinary practice**. It assesses the client's total situation and addresses the needs and problems found in that assessment. It is a means for improving client health, wellness, and autonomy. Case managers act within their profession and the boundaries of their competence, based on their education, skills, moral character, licensing and credentials, and experience. They recognize that everyone has the right to be treated with dignity and self-worth in obtaining quality services and cost-effective interventions and outcomes. Case managers provide advocacy, communication, and education, identify service resources, and facilitate services. Case managers recognize that case management is guided by the principles of autonomy, beneficence, nonmaleficence, and justice. Case managers strive to have the individual reach an optimum of wellness and functional capability benefiting the support systems, healthcare delivery systems, and the various reimbursement systems.

Key Domains of Case Management

The six key domains of case management include the following:

Domain	Description
Processes and Relationships	Encompass interpersonal relationships including communication and interviewing, case documentation, clinical problem-solving, negotiation, and conflict resolution.
Healthcare Management	Covers medical case management including aspects of acute and chronic illness and disability, the cost saving goals/objectives of case management, healthcare ethics, legal aspects of case management and clinical pharmacology.
Community Resources and Support	Requires knowledge of the various levels of care, community resources and support programs, rehabilitation services, and public benefit programs.
Service Delivery	Includes managed care and cost containment procedures, strategies and cost benefit analysis, healthcare benefits and delivery system, wellness concepts and strategies, case management models, and healthcare and disability-related legislation.
Psychosocial Intervention	Includes family dynamics, multicultural and neuropsychological assessment, mental health concepts, substance use/abuse/addiction, managed behavioral healthcare, and psychosocial aspects of chronic illness and disability
Rehabilitation Case Management	Includes disability compensation systems, job analysis/modification/accommodation, vocational assessment, job development and placement, ergonomics, and life-care planning.

Steps to Case Management

Managing a patient's care involves the following **steps**:

1. **Case finding happens through referrals:** Diagnosis-driven, high-dollar referrals or repeated service requests.
2. **Assessment** phase begins with the information that triggered the referral, contacting the patient if further action is warranted, obtaining signed consent forms, and establishing client rapport.
3. **Planning** includes contacting the patient's healthcare providers to obtain treatment plans, then developing the individualized plan.
4. **Reporting** includes desired outcomes, progress toward the outcomes, cost of care with and without case management and savings due to case management.
5. **Obtaining approval** requires documentation signed by the client (or their guardian).
6. **Coordination** means acting as liaison, coordinator, and communicator with everyone who is interested or plays a part in the case of the patient.
7. **Follow-up/monitoring** is a key component of the case manager's job. Ensuring that all providers and referrals send reports and updates is vital to maintaining the patient's records and preparing evaluations.
8. **Evaluation** is a dynamic function. The overall strategies and goals must be revised and evaluated after every patient contact and progress report.

Standards and Client Selection in Case Management

The following elements are considered standards of practice in case management:

- Client selection and assessment
- Problem/opportunity identification
- Planning, monitoring, and outcomes
- Termination of case management services
- Facilitation, coordination, and collaboration
- Qualifications for case managers
- Confidentiality and client privacy
- Consent for case management services
- Ethics and advocacy
- Cultural competency
- Resource management and stewardship
- Research and research utilization

The **client selection process** is one in which the case manager determines and selects clients who will receive the maximum benefit from the case management services that are available in a certain healthcare setting.

Identifying Potential Case Management Patients

Potential case management patients can be identified based on the following:

- Payers will often identify **catastrophic diagnosis** cases where complex, multiple care providers and services will be costly for both the patient and payer. These include HIV/AIDS, head injuries, neurological and back surgery, bone marrow transplants, etc.
- **High risk diagnoses** may lead to high-cost services. These include pregnancy induced hypertension, new onset seizure disorder, malignant cardiac arrhythmia, etc.
- Procedures that are associated with catastrophic diseases are called **sentinel procedures**. Case managers should review scheduling of these procedures. Some examples are major organ biopsies, arteriovenous shunt placement, and exploratory laparotomy.
- Any time an admitting diagnosis rises above the predetermined cost, the case manager should review the file. This is termed **high cost case selection** resulting from misleading or masked admitting diagnosis or unforeseen complications.
- **Passive case acquisitions** are received from requests for services from community members. The term "passive" refers to the fact that the case manager did not solicit the case and had no involvement in case selection. Direct case referral comes from established criteria and rules for case referrals.

Importance of Written Patient Records

Written patient records have the following features and benefits:

- They record the actions taken by case managers as well as the reasons for those actions.
- They provide the basis for reporting the costs and savings due to the use of case management.
- They allow others to manage the case in the absence of the assigned manager.
- They provide history and perspective for long and complex cases.
- They are necessary in the case of legal action to provide suitability of the care.

Remember that all conversations and information about a case fall within the **patient-provider privilege** and must follow disclosure rules.

Importance of Case Monitoring

Continued planning and **monitoring** takes into account changes in the client's health, living circumstances, and the success or failure of the links/transfer/referrals in the treatment plan. It is the case manager's responsibility to monitor the services provided to your client. The case manager must be certain the treatment or services authorized are being provided or used. All referrals should send reports at specified intervals. Referrals to informal (folk) support groups may require that the case manager contact them or provide a professional assessment to determine the success or failure of the services provided, as the group may not have the resources to provide the case manager with the information. Progress toward the goals in the individualized plan may need modifications or revisions or notations that goals were met. Reassessing the client allows adjustment of the timeline created in the initial assessment and restructuring of services needed. It provides the material needed to prepare a report on the success of case management, including all savings achieved.

Importance of a Life Care Plan

A life care plan is a comprehensive overview of the lifetime care of a patient based on clinical and financial information. A full analysis and narrative report of the current and future needs of a patient are included. Acquisition, replacement, repair and upgrading of medical services and items are included at current costs; a medical economist projects and adjusts them for inflation and financial trends. The life care plan is used in the court system as the groundwork for **settlements** in claims for personal injury or medical liability cases. The current and projected costs and utilization in the following areas must be included in the life care plan: financial status of the patient; medical, psychological, physical, and vocational rehabilitation; pharmaceutical and medical supply needs; social support resources; housing needs or architectural modifications; transportation needs; and prosthesis and assistive device needs.

Termination of Case Management Services

Termination of case management services is a standard of practice in case management. Appropriate termination of case management services is typically based upon established guidelines for case closure and will be different depending upon the practice setting of the case manager. Termination of case management may include the following reasons: the goal or maximum outcome has occurred, healthcare setting change, reduction or loss of healthcare benefits/eligibility, refusal of the client for further case management services, client noncompliance with the established healthcare plan, or death of the client. Termination of case management services may also occur with an agreement between the involved appropriate parties.

Case Management Tools

There are numerous tools and resources used in case management. Some examples include integration of three approaches to case management. The three approaches include the **individual care provider approach**, the **physician driven approach** that is based on treatment/critical pathways, and the **traditional discharge planning approach**. The most effective approach to case management combines all three approaches and utilizes tools and resources from the various approaches. Such case management tools may include gate-keeping screens to facilitate admission to the appropriate healthcare facility, critical pathways to guide minimally complex cases through the healthcare system, and variation analysis systems to study and guide the treatment of the more complex cases.

Case Management Models

Broker Model

The broker model of case management is also known as the broker service model, the generalist model, the standard model, and the traditional model. The broker model is designed to identify the needs of the client and to aid the client in the **access of the resources** that have been identified. Any form of case management planning may be limited and directed only to the client's initial contact with the case manager. Any form of continued monitoring is limited and typically does not include active advocacy. The somewhat limited relationship between the case manager and the client in this model allows the case manager to facilitate services to more clients.

Assertive Community Treatment Model

The assertive community treatment model of case management has an emphasis on the following areas:

- Contacting clients in their natural living environments
- Focusing upon the problems involved in the activities of daily living
- Demonstrating active and assertive advocacy
- Utilizing appropriate and manageable caseload size
- Implementing frequent and scheduled interactions between case manager and client
- Utilizing a team concept to share caseloads
- Maintaining long-term client involvement and commitment

The model of assertive community treatment also enables the case manager to provide more direct counseling to the client, to provide family consultations, to provide crisis interventions, and to act as facilitators in skill development.

Strengths-Based Model

The strengths-based model of case management is grounded in two principles. The first principle is that of **enabling** a client to gain personal control over the search for resources by providing support for finding housing and employment. The second principle is that of **analyzing** the strengths and assets that a client possesses as a means to obtain necessary resources. The strengths-based model of case management promotes the utilization of more informal resource networks as opposed to utilization of institutional networks. This model also places primary focus on the relationship between the case manager and the client and stresses aggressive and active client outreach.

Intensive Case Management Model

The intensive case management model is very similar to the assertive community treatment model, but there is a difference in the delivery of services. Intensive case management services are typically provided by an **individual case manager** as opposed to a case management team. Intensive case management involves a great deal more in case management than merely being a service brokerage. This model involves the establishment of a relationship between the case manager and the client and also stresses the provision of long-term support to the client to enable the client to function in an optimal manner and to improve quality of life.

Clinical Case Management Model

Clinical case management is defined by Kanter as "a modality of social work practice that, acknowledging the importance of biological and psychological factors, addresses the overall function and maintenance of the person's physical and social environment toward the goals of facilitating physical survival, health and mental health, personal growth, and community functioning." This model recognizes that clinical case management is a specialized and a professional field as opposed to just being a means of administering and coordinating services. The model of clinical case management also further stresses the necessity to integrate case management into a comprehensive **biopsychosocial treatment plan**.

Multidisciplinary Care Coordination Model

The multidisciplinary care coordination model focuses upon the proven fact that a quality healthcare system must have **continuity of care**. This model stresses the concept of a long-term relationship or partnership between the patient and healthcare providers that goes beyond just treatment of multiple episodes of illness and incorporates the responsibility for prevention and for care coordination. The multidisciplinary care coordination model has been shown to improve healthcare outcomes for patients and to decrease healthcare costs for complex medical conditions. The use of **electronic** medical records and electronic health information systems is essential in this model.

Demand Management Model

Demand management puts the burden of self-care on the patient. Case managers provide education avenues to patients but need to make sure they do not assist in determination of a diagnosis. Patients will be looking for confirmation of the conclusions they have drawn, and case managers need to avoid this discussion and make sure to fully document their discussions with patients.

Case managers must be aware of employers who use **carve-out programs** providing in-house resources (e.g., weight loss programs, on-site wellness activities). It is also important to know the employers utilizing **outsourcing** to achieve benefit oversight or customer service. The overseers of these carve-out programs and the outsource managers are contacts the case manager muse be aware of to provide assistance to their clients.

Levels of Care and Care Settings

Levels of Health Care

Various levels of health care exist to support specific conditions and populations.

Level of Care	Services Provided
Acute Care	Provides short-term medical treatments, usually in a hospital, for episodic illness or injury.
Long-Term Care	For major trauma patients or those with chronic and multiple medical, mental, and social problems who cannot take care of themselves.
Custodial Care	Assists clients with their home personal care and does not necessarily require the provider to have specialized skills or training.
Intermediate Care	For patients who require more than custodial care and might require nursing supervision. Unless true skilled care is required, insurance companies group intermediate and custodial care under the same benefit guidelines.
Skilled Nursing and Sub-Acute Care	For patients who need to be medically stable, requiring sub-acute rather than acute. Treatments in this level of care include frequent or complex wound care, rehabilitation, complex intravenous therapy, and combination therapies. Patients are usually in an extended care facility (ECF) such as a nursing home or a skilled nursing facility.

Transitional Hospitals

Transitional hospitals are acute care facilities for patients that are medically stable and whose rehabilitation plan is too complex for an **extended care facility (ECF)**. Transitional hospitals that specialize in medically complex care do so at a lower cost than a traditional hospital because of their specialization. Some transitional hospitals supply only basic patient care, also at a lower cost than a traditional hospital. Examples of transitional hospitals are: burn or extensive wound care, hemodialysis, hospice, infectious disease management, intravenous (IV) medication therapies, neurobehavioral rehabilitation, pain control therapies, rehabilitation, total parenteral nutrition, and ventilator care/weaning from ventilators.

Models of Care

Primary Nursing Model

There are numerous models of care in case management. The primary nursing model of care is an individualized and comprehensive model in which the same nurse gives care during the entire period of care. This method stresses care continuity and allows the nurse to provide direct patient care. The primary nurse has total 24-hour care responsibility for the patient. Such nursing care is oriented toward the goal of meeting the individualized needs of the patient. This model of primary nursing also utilizes the primary nurse to communicate with other members of the healthcare team regarding the patient's needs and total health care. Many institutions have rejected this care model as being cost prohibitive.

Case Management Model

The case management model of care originated in the 1990s. At that time, the model of nursing care was changed from a focus on quality of care to a focus on quality of care plus cost of care. This model of care was used extensively in social work and in outpatient psychiatry. The core of the case management model of care is the case management team. The case management team is an interdisciplinary group that convenes on a regular schedule to discuss and monitor a patient's health care and progress. Many consider this model to be cost effective in the current healthcare system.

Family-Centered Model

The family-centered model of care gained prominence in the healthcare field at the end of the twentieth century. The family-centered model recognized that the family is usually the center of a patient's life and that the family usually is often expert in the knowledge of a patient's abilities and needs. This model enables the family to collaborate with the healthcare providers in helping the patient make informed decisions about healthcare services and supports. Strengths and weaknesses of all the family members are often also considered in this model of care. This model of care has resulted in increased patient satisfaction.

Public Health Nursing Model

The public health nursing model of care is based upon the idea that public health care is population based. This model of care primarily focuses on an entire population that has similar health issues. The public health model of care also focuses on the broad scope of the determinants of health. Public health care targets all levels of prevention, with its primary focus being that of **primary prevention. Secondary prevention** is an additional focus in the public healthcare model, and it tries to detect and treat healthcare problems in earlier stages. This model also focuses on tertiary prevention to hopefully prevent existing healthcare issues from worsening.

Integrative Model

The integrative model of care is sometimes referred to as the **interdisciplinary model of care**. This model of care involves cooperation and communication between a team of healthcare professionals. Information sharing among such professionals allows for the development of a comprehensive treatment plan that encompasses the medical, psychological, and social needs of a patient. The integrative health team may include physicians, nurses, social workers, psychologists, and occupational/physical therapists. Such a coordinated model of care can improve quality of life, decrease healthcare costs, and provide a positive benefit to patients over their lifespan. This model of care may also include a focus on the holistic or "whole-person" aspects of a patient's care.

Medical Home Model

The medical home model is a healthcare approach to providing care (primary and comprehensive) to patients. This healthcare model serves to coordinate and improve relationships between patients, their families, and their personal physicians. In March 2007, the American Academy of Family Physicians, American Academy of Pediatrics, American College of Physicians, and American Osteopathic Association developed **joint principles** for the medical home model. The characteristics of these principles are a personal physician, physician-directed medical practice, focus on the whole person, coordinated care, focus on quality and safety of medical care, enhanced patient access, and payment.

Chronic Care Model

According to the CDC about 133 million Americans are impacted by chronic disease, and approximately 40 million are limited in their usual activities due to chronic disease. The chronic care model was developed to manage patients with chronic medical conditions in a proactive manner as opposed to the traditional reactive manner. This model integrates the basic components for improving medical care in health systems at numerous levels. These levels of health systems are the **community**, the **organization**, the **provider practice**, and the **patient**. There are three basic themes in the chronic care model. The model is **evidence-based**, **population-based**, and **patient-centered**. The theme of evidence-based stresses the importance of evidence and excellence as opposed to autonomy.

Tools of Chronic Care Model

The six tools of the chronic care model are decision support, clinical information systems, delivery system design, the healthcare organization, community resources and policies, and self-management support. **Decision support systems** are utilized to facilitate the use of the best available evidence and to apply such evidence to clinical decision making. Evidence-based guidelines are incorporated into medical care. **Clinical information systems** can be electronic only or can be a mixture of electronic and paper. A vital component of a clinical information system is a registry. A registry is a clinical information tool that may track an individual patient or a patient population base.

Delivery System and Healthcare Organization

Components of a successful delivery system design in the chronic care model include an emphasis on the concept of team care with the roles and job tasks of each member defined. The healthcare team schedules visits or meetings to integrate evidence-based medicine with ongoing chronic care. The delivery system design gives healthcare management to high-risk patients and emphasizes regular follow-up and ongoing care coordination. It also provides centralized and current information on patient status. The **healthcare organization** promotes improved quality assurance through information, education, incentives, and frequent or ongoing evaluations.

Self-Management

Self-management in the chronic care model is not the same as telling a patient what to do. Effective self-management in this model involves interventions, constant cooperative goal setting, and problem solving by the healthcare team. There are five basic "A's" in self-management in the chronic care model:

Assess	the knowledge, confidence, and behaviors on a routine basis.
Advise	the patient and the team using scientific evidence and current information.
Agree	upon goals and treatment.
Assist	the patient to identify problems and barriers.
Arrange	services.

Lifespan Considerations

Differentiating Care Based on Age

The case manager must differentiate care based on age:

- **Pediatrics**: The needs of caregivers (usually parents) for support and education/training must be considered as well as the availability of community resources. In addition to health concerns, the case manager must consider the child's need for recreation, stimulation, and education.
- **Adults**: Focus is on educating the client about healthcare, managing illness, and dealing with psychosocial issues, such as changes in relationships and loss of income resulting from illness. Clients may require different types of services, such as social workers and physical and vocational rehabilitation.
- **Older adults**: Concerns include caregiver stress as well as client needs, such as managing chronic disease, assessing cognitive ability, and reducing hospitalizations. Clients often have multiple healthcare providers and multiple medications. Focus is often on functional ability and whether the client can live independently or needs supportive care. Clients may need increased reminders regarding treatments and appointments.

Additional Lifespan Considerations

The case manager must be aware of the needs specific to different points in the lifespan of clients. Specific considerations include:

- **Individualized care**: Each client should be assessed for needs, which may vary by age and over time, and a care plan should be developed.
- **Safety concerns**: For children, education regarding safety focuses on the parents/guardians, and later on the client and/or caregivers. Environmental modifications and safety needs vary over time.
- **Community resources**: Needed resources may vary widely. Children may, for example need educational programs and financial assistance for parents/guardians while adults may need transportation and meal services as well as home health care. Older adults may need assistance with personal care and/or assisted living.
- **Medication management**: Parents/Guardians and clients may need education about medications and treatments. Older adults are especially at risk for polypharmacy.
- **Crisis prevention/intervention**: Parents/Guardians of children and caregivers for adults are especially at risk of burnout and may require support and time out in order to provide adequate care for clients. Children may resist treatments, especially during adolescence, and adults may become increasingly depressed and stressed with chronic illness.

Case Management and Population Health

Case management increasingly focuses not only on the needs of the individual but also on population health and the needs of specific groups, such as those with chronic disease (heart failure, hypertension, trauma, chest pain, COPD, HIV, sickle cell disease, chronic pain) or age-delineated groups (pediatrics, adolescents, adults, older adults). The role of the case manager is to coordinate population services (screening, education, assessment, smoking cessation programs), assess population needs, and establish interventions to improve compliance with treatment and to reduce emergency department visits, hospitalizations, and lengths of stay. The case manager may develop a risk assessment program to determine target interventions as well as clinical pathways to serve as a guide for others in providing care. The case manager must incorporate methods of disease prevention and health promotion, focusing on education of the target population to inform and motivate members of the population to establish goals, adopt healthy habits, and make lifestyle changes.

Alternative Care Facilities

Group Homes

Group homes are considered a type of alternative care facility. Typically, a group home is small, residential, and it functions to care for patients with chronic disabilities. These group homes are usually small and have six or fewer residents. Group homes are staffed around the clock by trained personnel. The typical group home is a single-family residence that is paid for by the group home administrators. It is usually adapted to meet the special needs of its patients. Group home residents may have chronic mental or physical disabilities that require assistance or supervision or aid with the activities of daily living.

Residential Treatment Facilities

Another alternative care facility is a residential treatment facility. Resident treatment facilities may also be referred to as **rehab facilities**. Residential treatment facilities serve as a live-in situation in which therapies for substance abuse, behavioral issues, and mental illness are provided. Residential treatment facilities may be either locked or unlocked. **Locked facilities** are quite restrictive and may confine the patient to a single room or cell. **Unlocked residential treatment facilities** generally afford the patient much more freedom in the facility, but there are certain conditions/supervision required in order to leave the facility. In general, most residential treatment facilities are of a clinical focus and often utilize behavior modification techniques.

Assisted Living Facilities

Assisted living facilities are also considered a type of alternative care facility. Assisted living is designed to aid community residents with the activities of daily living. Some state regulations will allow an assisted living facility to provide assistance or reminders for medications. Assisted living facilities are different from nursing homes in that such facilities do not provide complex medical services. Assisted living communities vary from a stand-alone facility to being one tier of care in a continuing care retirement facility. Usually, the assisted living environment is more like a personal home or apartment. The cost for an assisted living facility is usually paid via private funds; however, some exceptions exist. Some long-term-care insurance policies provide for such fees; Medicaid and waivers may also be available.

Home Care Services

Common alternatives to hospital treatment are rehabilitation and skilled nursing facilities. The newest alternative is **home care**, one of today's fastest growing industries, providing services by licensed/certified personnel in a setting that contributes to faster recovery, a better quality of life and decreased risk of contracting a **nosocomial illness** (an illness from a hospital-borne infection), all at substantial cost savings over formal facility care. Home care is not for acutely ill individuals needing specialized programs or skilled nursing facilities. The family situation needs to be able to support the needs of the patient (treatment and medication schedules) without making them feel like a burden. Children improve quicker in a home setting with fewer lingering psychological issues. Technology has made it feasible to use home care for patients needing dialysis, blood transfusions, ventilators or pain management, as well long-term illnesses such as AIDS, brain injury, or chronic neurological problems (multiple sclerosis) or those that are terminally ill. For patients recuperating from surgery, it is important to have a coordinated team approach to ensure that quality, comprehensive services are provided.

Role of Case Managers

Coordination of services for home care is an important function of case management. Assuring the patient and family that home care is a viable, safe option is of primary importance. Then a visit to the home ensures home care can be accommodated. Liability for providing appropriate care is a function of all personnel involved in the patient's treatment plan; however, the discharging primary care physician must provide the sign off on discharge orders. The case manager must devise a home care plan that meets all criteria of the discharge plan. The patient's family and community resources, geographical location and availability of health care and durable medical equipment providers as well as emergency services must be taken into account. Depending on the circumstances, case managers may need to make a case for coverage to the insurance carrier with cost savings as the primary benefit.

Importance of Case Management

Home care is an area that requires detailed **monitoring** and **documentation** by case managers. Any deficiencies in performance of services by recommended vendors reflect on the case manager and are subject to legal action. Input about vendor performance from the patient and caregiver is important to obtain on a regular basis. The case manager must be aware of changing needs of the patient and make sure they are reflected in the care plan. The patient's adherence to the care plan and successes or failures must be noted and adjustments made to the care plan to meet any changes. Caregiver psychological and physical well-being must also be noted and respite care investigated. Intervention with payers may be needed to cover respite care and the real threat of covering the costs of the caregiver's breakdown is a compelling reason. It is important for the case manager to remember that their negotiation skills in obtaining cost effective services is the key to home health care savings. Their ability to negotiate with the payer is also key in assuring that the cost of home care will result in overall cost savings and thus be covered by the insurance plan, especially if a variance in coverage is needed.

Problems

Home care is not without drawbacks. The home must be able to accommodate the durable equipment needed and provide a safe environment for the patient for both recovery and treatment activities. A **safe environment** begins with the cleanliness of the home and the ability of the family to provide nourishment and cleanliness needed for healing. Often caregivers need to use physical exertion to move patients. This can cause complications for the caregiver as well as create an unsafe environment for the patient. The patient must have an environment that will allow healing and not make them feel like they are a burden to the caregiver*Case managers must be cognizant throughout the case of stress on the caregiver and the family and the resulting effect on the patient.

Resources

Home care is available from a variety of sources. **Skilled professionals** in nursing and therapy fields are available through private sources, however cost savings are available by exploring **alternative providers**. Local, county or state agencies support a variety of professional services delivered in the home (e.g., visiting nurses association) or available at their facility on a day-visit basis (e.g., senior day care or dialysis). Disease-specific organizations (childhood diabetes), foundations and non-profit groups (Shriner's burn center) are also sources for home care support. Some of these same organizations offer respite care enabling the patient to spend up to a week away from home enabling the caregiver to "recharge."

Assessing Practicality

Home care is the fastest growing component of healthcare due to the **viability** of even complex care being handled in the home (e.g., ventilators, total parenteral nutrition, or infusion care). The case manager must look at the medical, financial, and social situation of the patient to determine if home care is a viable option. Managed care has spearheaded the home care alternative and Medicare has allowed the care with contracts with health maintenance organizations (HMOs). The case manager must review the patient's insurance coverage benefits for the necessary treatments before recommending home care versus facility care. Traditionally the following criteria must be met for **home health visits**:

- The patient is confined to their home or has great difficulty going to an outpatient facility.
- The care requires intermittent skilled nursing services and may include physical, occupational and speech therapies.
- The patient's care plan is reasonable, medically necessary, and overseen by a physician who reviews the care plan at least every 60 days.
- The home healthcare agency is Medicare-certified, meeting the strictest federal standards.

Telehealth

Telehealth refers to the delivery of healthcare services to patients who are not physically present with the healthcare professional, usually due to remote location, disability, or pandemic (such as the recent outbreak of COVID-19). Telehealth can be delivered over a telephone, via email, or by video conference. The primary benefits of telehealth are that it allows for the extension of precious healthcare resources, lowers the overall cost of healthcare, and allows patients to receive healthcare who would not normally have access to it.

There are a number of **ways in which telehealth is useful** to healthcare professionals:

- Consultation with colleagues
- Patient interviews and monitoring
- Monitor a patient's biometric values and assess their condition
- Evaluate diagnostic images which allows physicians to remotely view and evaluate these images even if they are located overseas (e.g., India)
- Evaluation of microscope slides and laboratory reports

Cost Containment and Financial Resources

Cost Containment Principles

The rapidly rising costs of health care need to be curtailed; the system is now focusing on attaining better outcomes while controlling costs. Over- and underutilization of services in health care is one principle in **cost containment**. Improved coordination and cooperation over the entire quality of care continuum is another principle. Another principle is placing greater emphasis upon prevention by awarding incentives for wellness behaviors in patients as well as stressing early detection of disease. Increased usage of evidence-based guidelines in the treatment of various diseases helps to contain costs. Electronic medical records and improved information regarding the costs of products and services used by providers and patients allow informed decisions about the comparative effectiveness of treatments.

Extra-Contractual Benefit Plans

Insurance plans can have **limitations** or **exclusions** that may hinder the most efficient and cost-effective medical care. Case managers may see cost reduction benefits in care that would not be covered under the patient's insurance plan. Case managers need to prepare a report clearly stating the benefits and cost reductions in allowing **extra-contractual benefits**. They need to communicate with the insurer and obtain approval by the payer and knowledge of the approval received by the claims adjuster, prior to the implementation of the care/program. Obtaining extra-contractual benefits is one part of maximizing resources at the patient's disposal.

Pros and Cons of Capitation

Capitation is a fee scenario where the provider and managed care organization predict the expenses and revenue of a population group then set a rate for the number of lives covered rather than the services provided. The provider receives a set amount of money each month based on the number of patients in the program, not the number seen for services. The provider purchases reinsurance or stop-loss insurance to cover catastrophic cases. Capitation is seen as a means of cost control, focusing on preventative services to identify early and reduce the expense of catastrophic illness. Criticism of capitation is aimed at physicians who will/do not refer patients for extensive tests or under-treat patients. Physicians may also focus more on fee-for-service patients, which causes patients to question the motivation of the physician to properly treat them. Regulatory and licensing issues have been raised since physicians are acting as the insurer. Capitation has demonstrated a decrease in the need and cost of specialty services. It has increased the availability of preventative services and early detection of disease while stopping physicians from over-treating patients. It enhances a physician's cash flow.

Managed Care Organizations

Managed care is a financial system developed as a cost containment system in the healthcare industry. Managed care organizations (MCO) have a case manager who oversees the care given a patient in order to prevent costs from running over the amount allocated for the disease/treatment. An MCO case manager may need to provide pre-authorization for hospital admittance or for treatment options of clients with developmental disabilities, substance abuse problems or mental health issues. Managed care is an economic system and thus could be at odds with the individualized plan for your client, or the MCO may require their case manager be the only case manager for your client.

Managed Competition

Managed Care Organization (MCO) is a generic term that is used to describe many types of medical care plans including HMO, PPO, IPA, etc. California's 1993 reforms for workers' compensation claims saw the creation of health care organizations (HCOs) to apply MCO principles to work-related injuries. As managed care evolves, dental care providers are creating managed care networks. **Managed competition** is the term given to the business environment created by the managed care entities competing for business. Many large companies are negotiating discount arrangements from healthcare and prescription providers, durable medical equipment supplies or rehabilitation facilities. A case manager must be aware of the mergers taking place between providing companies to assure quality of care and the effects of business relationships on their ability to negotiate on behalf of their client. The case manager may also be limited in the offerings they can present in the individualized plan due to arrangements between the insurer and healthcare providers.

Waiver Programs

Waiver programs are those developed by states to test new ways to deliver services for Medicaid and Children's Health Insurance Program (CHIP). The four primary types of waivers include:

- **Research and demonstration projects**: Allow flexibility in program design.
- **Managed care**: Services may limit patient's choices.
- **Home and community-based services**: Long-term care services provided in the home and community rather than in institutions.
- **Concurrent**: Involves two types of waivers used to provide continuum of services for older adults and the disabled.

Case management services that may be covered under the waivers include reviewing service plans annually, assisting patients to identify and access healthcare providers, coordinating services, developing and monitoring a plan of care, and providing information to the patient or patient's representative regarding service options. Administrative activities are not billable under waivers. All billable services must be actually provided to the patient and not based on averages.

Viatical Settlements

A case manager works with many people who are terminally ill or draining their finances in order to cope with an illness. A **viatical settlement** is a means of obtaining a portion of the cash value of a life insurance policy before the covered individual's death. In a viatical settlement, an investment company pays the covered individual a significant percentage of the death benefit immediately and assumes responsibility for all future premium payments in exchange for being named as the beneficiary of the policy. The percentage that is paid to the individual depends primarily on life expectancy but is usually in the 50-85% range. Life insurance companies may also be willing to negotiate an early payout of a similar portion of the death benefit if the individual is terminally ill.

Non-Traditional Policies

Non-traditional or supplemental policies provide comprehensive coverage for a wide range of treatments. These policies include disease-specific policies, such as those covering cancer or Alzheimer's; long-term care or nursing home policies; occupation-specific policies (e.g., a model or an athlete insuring their hands/legs); as well as Medigap, dental, and vision policies.

Special Needs Trusts

Special needs trusts are set up so that disabled individuals can receive financial assistance without it affecting their eligibility for SSI or Medicaid. The trust cannot pay money directly to the beneficiary but can pay for goods and services, such as medical expenses, recreation, education, supplies, and furniture. In some cases, pooled trusts are set up with multiple family members contributing. Special needs trusts may be first person trusts (set up by the beneficiary with money originating from the beneficiary, such as from an inheritance) or third person trusts (set up by someone else for the beneficiary). Third party trusts are commonly set up in a will or living trust in order to provide ongoing support for an individual after a caregiver dies and does not take effect until after the death of the benefactor. If the support is to be provided before the benefactor dies, this is a stand-alone trust. If the trust is irrevocable, the eligibility is preserved for SSI and Medicaid, but if the trust is revocable, the assets must be considered for eligibility.

End-of-Life Care

End-of-Life Issues

End-of-life issues may include adequate pain control, avoidance of prolonged suffering and a prolonged dying process, adequate discussion with the patient and family members, a sense of control, appropriate preparation for death with a sense of completion, reinforcing relationships, and a sense of not being alone. End-of-life care may utilize hospice. **Hospice** is a holistic approach that utilizes the entire care team to make the dying patient as comfortable as possible and stresses pain control, natural death, and the quality of life that is remaining. **Palliative care** stresses symptom management and relief from pain. **Drug therapy** is common, but alternative methods may also be used, including acupuncture, massage therapy, and aromatherapy. **Do not resuscitate (DNR)** is a legal order that recognizes the choice of a patient to not undergo cardiopulmonary resuscitation (CPR)/advanced cardiac life support (ACLS) and to die a natural death; this order basically does not affect any treatment other than that which may necessitate intubation or CPR. DNR patients may still receive chemotherapy, dialysis, antibiotics, and other therapies.

Case Manager's Role in End-of-Life

Although death is inevitable, more than 50% of Americans 45 years or older have never discussed end of life (EOL) issues with their families, including thoughts about death when someone was terminally ill. Case managers have the unique position to be able to assist individuals and their families with fact-based information and alleviate their fears. It is important for case managers to know the laws in the state in which they practice. The **Patient Self-Determination Act (PSDA)** of 1991 requires all Medicare and Medicaid agencies to recognize living wills and powers of attorney for advanced directives in healthcare; however, states have their own definitions and practices regarding guarantees for individual rights to determine treatment. **Do not resuscitate (DNR) orders, living wills, healthcare proxies** (wishes regarding life-prolonging measures), and other legal documents are areas where case managers make an impact on the treatment their clients will receive. These advance directives assist families during crisis situations by allowing discussion and decisions to be made in advance.

Palliative Care

Palliative care is defined by the World Health Organization as "an approach that improves the quality of life of patients and their families facing problems associated with life-limiting illness, through the prevention of suffering by means of early identification and impeccable assessment and treatment of pain and other problems, physical, psychological, and spiritual." Such palliative care encompasses a **holistic approach** to health care that may include measures to facilitate physical, psychological, spiritual, and social well-being for the patient. Importantly, the family and significant others of the patient are also involved and included in the palliative care process.

Principles of Symptom Management

Multiple symptoms may present in a patient who is receiving palliative care, and they require careful management. Such symptoms may include severe pain, fatigue, anorexia, nausea, vomiting, weakness, dry mouth, and dyspnea. **Symptom management principles in palliative care** may include taking an aggressive and detailed approach to identifying and prioritizing symptoms. Symptom management may be pharmacological or nonpharmacological in nature.

- **Pharmacological symptom management** needs to focus on the underlying cause or causes of the symptoms. For example, nausea may be a side effect of prescribed medications, chemotherapy, or a possible bowel obstruction.
- **Nonpharmacological symptom management** may include alternative medicine such as acupuncture, aromatherapy, or massage.

Hospice Care

Hospice is a healthcare program that provides support and comfort to patients and families dealing with the final stages of terminal illness. The goal is to provide care at home, although specialized hospice facilities exist in many locations. **Medicare** covers hospice care if ALL of the following apply:

- A physician certifies the patient is terminally ill with 6 months or less to live.
- The patient or family requests hospice assistance.
- The provider is Medicare-certified.

The physician's hospice referral can be made from either a home or hospital setting. To receive hospice care coverage, a patient must **waive** standard Medicare benefits for the illness/condition causing the hospice referral; however, care for other conditions unrelated to the hospice referral condition are covered by standard Medicare benefits. Medicare Part A pays for two 90-day and unlimited 60-day benefit periods, with recertification being subject to a doctor's (or nurse practitioner's) re-evaluation of the patient.

Respite Care

Respite care is the psychological and physical support provided to caregivers of those with chronic disease. Respite care takes many forms. Especially in cases involving long-term care, caregivers need to be encouraged to talk with others in similar situations, facing similar challenges by attending caregiver support groups. To better understand illnesses, support services are available for spouses, children, siblings, and other family members of individuals suffering from long-term illnesses. Respite care may be in the form of camp for a child suffering from an illness (cancer, diabetes) allowing the family to be free of responsibility for the time the patient is away. Respite care may be placement of an elderly person at an assisted living residence for a weekend giving the family care providers a "weekend off." Respite care may be someone residing in the home of a patient allowing the family caregivers to take a vacation. Case managers can assist by identifying when caregivers need respite care and by supplying resources for respite care.

Interdisciplinary Care

Interdisciplinary Care Team

Theresa Drinka defines the interdisciplinary care team as "a group of individuals with diverse training and backgrounds who work together as an identified unit or system. Team members consistently collaborate to solve patient problems that are too complex to be solved by one discipline or many disciplines in sequence. In order to provide care as efficiently as possible, an interdisciplinary care team creates **formal and informal structures** that encourage collaborative problem solving. Team members determine the team's mission and common goals; work interdependently to define and treat patient problems; and learn to accept and capitalize on disciplinary differences, differential power, and overlapping roles. To accomplish these goals, they share leadership that is appropriate to the presenting problem and promote the use of differences for confrontation and collaboration."

Advantages

There are many advantages to an interdisciplinary care team. In this approach, the patient is more actively engaged in the healthcare decision-making process as a result of the team of being patient centered. Another major advantage to the interdisciplinary care team is that such teams foster an environment in which diverse specialties may learn from one another. Interdisciplinary care teams also have the advantages of being more efficient and cost-effective. These advantages are manifested by eliminating duplication of services and by eliminating the necessity of case conferencing follow-up. Lastly, clinical information sharing in an interdisciplinary care team reduces medical errors.

Management of Clients with Illness

Disease Management vs. Case Management

Case management oversees an individual patient, whereas **disease management** focuses on groups of patients with diagnostic conditions that historically have high financial costs and will benefit from integrated and systematic management of treatment. The goal of disease management is to reach individuals at the earliest possible time in the disease cycle. Assessment of the patient in relation to the disease's risks allows planning and intervention services at appropriate times to reduce both the chronic nature of the disease and the cost complications. The following diseases are among those that have demonstrated the effectiveness of disease management: diabetes, asthma, cardiovascular disease, multiple sclerosis, and arthritis. Only through patient interviews will it be determined if an individual needs disease management.

Focuses of Disease Management

Disease management, or condition management, focuses on **populations** with widespread, often chronic, diseases with varying care practices. Non-disease conditions, such as pregnancy or cessation of smoking, are also candidates for disease/condition management. Participants are identified via claims review, new member health assessments or provider referrals. Disease management allows knowledge to be transferred among the population and care providers. Case managers may be assigned responsibility to communicate with participants in disease/condition management programs sending out information or informing participants of educational opportunities. Just as in case management, disease management resources should be documented and the savings of using sound management processes should be calculated and reported.

Multiple Comorbidities

Case management is a vital step in the care of patients with multiple comorbidities. Some successful strategies for management include customizing care for an individual patient, coordinated hospital discharge planning and counseling, intensive care coordination between multiple providers and the patient, frequent personal contact with the patient, early physician involvement, careful follow-up, involvement of multidisciplinary teams that provide treatment and patient support such as nutrition, pharmacy, and social services, ease of access to healthcare providers to prevent exacerbations, home visits post-hospital-discharge, patient education, and telephone contact with the patient on a frequent basis.

HIV/AIDS Management

Around 1.2 million people in the US were affected by HIV as of 2018, with nearly 40,000 new cases annually. It is a disease of the immune system that allows other diseases to invade the body. The spread of HIV/AIDS is due to risky behavior (primarily sexual activity and drug/needle sharing), drug resistance, treatment noncompliance, and denial. Approximately 40% of HIV/AIDS patients also have hepatitis C, which also requires aggressive treatment. Because AIDS compromises the immune system, complications and coexisting conditions are frequent. AIDS clients require **long-term care case management** and increased awareness of confidentiality, social stigmatization, prejudice, and manipulation of benefits. Barriers and roadblocks are often encountered in trying to coordinate treatments and resources for AIDS patients. Due to confidentiality, benefits may be denied based on a diagnostic code, and the case manager may need to be proactive to resolve the issues. Case managers need to empower AIDS clients to take an active role in the management of their treatment. The patient is the first to recognize changes, and communication with their case manager allows realignment of the treatment plan.

Review Video: AIDS Infections and Malignancies
Visit mometrix.com/academy and enter code: 319526

Case Manager Preparation

It is important for case managers to examine their **beliefs and feelings about death** before handling AIDS cases. It is important not to pre-judge the patient based on their AIDS diagnosis. Understanding AIDS and the diseases associated with AIDS is important in providing services to the patient. Knowing community resources and educational sources including Internet sites are important aspects of managing AIDS cases and assisting the patient in self-management of their treatment. Understanding their own feelings about death will enable the case manager to **cope** with the loss of an AIDS patient. The case manager needs to be prepared to cope with the inevitable death of the patient, someone who shared intimate details of their life or their thoughts about suicide due to the physical degradation they will suffer. Conversely, the case manager may need to deal with someone in denial of their demise. It is important for the case manager to avoid painting a positive picture of the outcome of the treatment plan, a view contrary to the case manager's usual patient interaction. The case manager may need to identify their own **support mechanism** while handling AIDS cases.

Drug Therapy and Lifestyle Changes

The title *case manager* implies **management** not **monitoring**. In handling HIV/AIDS cases, it is important for case managers to inquire about new therapies and drug interactions and obtain research information about the disease. Advances in antiretroviral drug and protease inhibitor combinations (triple cocktails), along with an understanding of the effects of nutrition and supplements, has moved HIV infections into chronic disease, long-term care. Case managers can stress wellness and prevention strategies in the treatment plans as well as including return-to-work scenarios. The key to surviving with HIV is early diagnosis and starting therapy, use of viral load indicators and CD4+ T-cell counts, aggressive treatments using a minimum of 3 drugs, recognition and identification of opportunistic infections and protein-calorie malnutrition, restoration of the immune system, understanding mind-body connection, and empowering the HIV-infected person to assume self-management. Assisting the individual in understanding the importance of maintaining body weight (adds 10 years) is another key factor in stopping HIV from advancing to AIDS. The disease consumes calories. A 10% reduction of body weight reduces life expectancy and over 30% of patients die from "wasting syndrome."

Triple Cocktails

Triple cocktails are combinations of antiretroviral drugs that reduce HIV virus levels. Reduction of the virus to below detection level reduces the incidence of opportunistic diseases and slows other signs of the disease's progression. Drug treatments are expensive ($12,000-$15,000/year) and must be ingested in a specific sequence within a specific time period. The administration of the drugs presents a challenge to patients and caregivers; the drugs have debilitating **side effects** and affect different patients in different ways and are only effective in 30% of patients, in part due to the difficulty in administering the drugs. Case managers need to be aware of **toxicity** and **resistance** issues with HIV patients. The drugs compete with one another causing reactions and they also interact with foods to cause side effects. Protease inhibitors can cause metabolic upheaval such as maldistribution of body fat resulting in a disproportional look. HIV drugs can cause adverse interactions in combination with over-the-counter and certain prescription drugs. Case managers need to be aware of **harmful drug interactions**. Assisting patients in researching and obtaining drugs through free distribution programs, direct from manufacturers or becoming part of research studies is an important role for case managers.

Prevention Case Management

Prevention case management (PCM) links clients with the services they need, providing coordination and brokerage of services beyond what the client might be able to obtain without the benefit of a case manager. For persons living with HIV, **coordination** needs to exist between health care, psychiatric, psychosocial, and other community support services. For clients with HIV, there needs to be **identification** of risk behaviors and development of a prevention plan that outlines specific behavioral objectives. Part of the medical and psychosocial services includes STD evaluation and treatment and substance abuse treatment. The goal of HIV primary prevention is reduction of the transmission and acquisition of HIV infection. The goal of HIV secondary prevention is to prevent a person with HIV from becoming ill or dying as a result of HIV-related illness. HIV prevention case management requires **community understanding and support**. It is important to understand the norms, values and traditions sanctioned by the community leaders and accepted by the population in order to succeed in PCM. In other words, the case manager must have cultural competence.

Heart Disease Management

The case manager must employ a number of strategies in case management of patients with heart disease. The case manager should engage the patient in planning and should coordinate care. Goals of care often include improving the quality of life and functional ability, so this may require referral to physical therapy and occupational therapy. Patients often benefit from **cardiac care programs** that assist the patient in developing an exercise program and understanding diet needs. Patients with heart disease require frequent monitoring and follow-up to ensure that they receive recommended healthcare services and adhere to prescribed diet and medications. A primary challenge in case management of patients with heart disease is that many patients are older adults who may be frail and live alone or with an older spouse. Patients may lack adequate income for medications and treatment and may lack health literacy.

Stroke Management

The case manager must employ a number of strategies in case management of patients with strokes. Goals include:

- **Maximal physical recovery**: This may include referral to PT, OT, and speech therapy as well as treatment in a rehabilitation center. Recovery may be a lengthy process; however, patients are often older adults with limited resources. Many live alone or with elderly spouses or reluctant family caregivers, so ongoing participation in recovery efforts is often limited. Referral to a social worker is often needed.
- **Hypertension control**: Patients often have lifestyle choices (poor diet, lack of exercise, smoking, drinking) that increase BP. Patients may benefit from smoking- or drinking-cessation programs and diet instruction. They may need education about the importance of adherence to medications and plan of care.
- **Fall prevention**: Stroke patients are at risk of falls, so an environmental assessment prior to discharge is important, , but patients may lack the motivation or financial resources necessary to make environmental changes necessary for safety.

Review Video: Overview of Strokes
Visit mometrix.com/academy and enter code: 310572

Difficulties

The case manager faces a number of common difficulties in assisting a patient post-stroke to transition to the next level of care. If a patient is transitioning to a rehabilitation center or extended care facility, the primary difficulty lies in communication. The **discharge summary** must be complete and should thoroughly outline the patient's condition, treatment, and plan of care. The case manager should communicate directly with healthcare providers at the transfer organization. If a patient is transitioning to the home, then family members or caregivers must be involved in the planning process and should be educated about fall prevention and patient needs. The patient often faces numerous emotional, social, and environmental problems, including access to the home. These issues may best be assessed through referral to a social worker and home health agency. The patient may need ongoing PT, OT, and speech therapy. Patients often fail to adhere to the plan of care and stop taking medications, so **ongoing support** is critical.

Obesity Management

The case manager should take a proactive role in case management of patients with obesity, first by ensuring that all patients be screened for obesity, which can be accomplished through BMI and waist circumference. **Obesity screens** assist in assessing risks. Controlling obesity may improve outcomes for chronic disease and serve as a preventive measure. The case manager should review patient's **medications** to determine those that may contribute to weight gain, such as corticosteroids. The case manager may encourage **behavioral treatment**, utilizing motivational interviewing to help overcome resistance, and should include techniques for self-monitoring and stimulus control. The obese patient must be educated about food and diet and may benefit from referral to a nutritionist. Maintaining a food diary or participating in a weight loss program, such as Weight Watchers, may help patients maintain good eating habits. Patients should begin a program of physical exercise to tolerance, and the case manager should monitor progress. The case manager and other healthcare providers should provide emotional support to the patient because many patients lose weight only to promptly regain it.

Cancer Management

The case manager faces many challenges in caring for patients with cancer, especially those with advanced disease who require difficult treatments, such as surgery, radiation therapy, and chemotherapy. The case manager must coordinate aspects of the patient's care, maintaining effective communication with all healthcare providers. Patient needs may include:

- **Social needs**: Patients may need assistance with transportation, meal preparation, finances, and family interactions. Referral to social workers is often indicated.
- **Health/Treatment needs**: Patients must be monitored to ensure that they receive medical treatment and palliative care as needed, including methods of reducing pain and managing nausea and vomiting. Patients may benefit from home health care. Patients may have various co-morbidities, such as heart disease or diabetes, which must be attended to as well.
- **Fear and anxiety**: Patients may need referral to cancer support groups or may need counseling or other support services.
- **Hospice care**: The case manager should ensure the patient is provided information about hospice when appropriate and help the patient transition from active treatment to hospice care.

Diabetes Management

The patient with diabetes requires attention from the case manager in a number of different areas when coordinating the plan of care:

- **Co-morbidities/Complications**: Patients with diabetes may have a number of co-morbidities, such as heart disease and arthritis, and these may result in the need to modify standard treatment plans. Patients may have poor vision or neuropathy that interferes with their ability to manage their disease.
- **Self-management**: Both patients and family members/caregivers must receive information about the disease and preventive measures, such as controlling hypertension, carrying out good skin care, and maintaining proper diet. They also need education regarding administration of medications (oral anti-glycemic agents and/or insulin) and monitoring of condition (blood glucose, Hgb A1c).
- **Behavioral/Lifestyle modification**: Patients may need assistance in weight loss, smoking and/or drinking cessation as well as eating and exercise habits.
- **Psychosocial needs**: Patients often need emotional support and may lack the financial resources or transportation needed to manage their disease and follow through with monitoring. Referral to social workers may be needed.

Review Video: Diabetes Mellitus: Complications
Visit mometrix.com/academy and enter code: 996788

Review Video: Diet, Exercise, and Medications for Diabetes
Visit mometrix.com/academy and enter code: 774388

Arthritis Management

The case manager's involvement with patients with arthritis may vary depending on the type of arthritis and the degree of physical impairment. Issues that are common with arthritis patients include:

- **Organization of care**: Patients may require PT and OT and various treatments, such as DMARDs or surgery, from a variety of healthcare providers; and treatment must be scheduled and preauthorized as needed.
- **Patient education**: Patients and family/caregivers may need education about medications, treatment, and preventive measures in order to understand and make informed decisions.
- **Functional ability/Pain**: Patients may have varying degrees of physical limitations and may require environmental modification and assistive devices. Pain control is often an ongoing problem that requires assistance.
- **Medication/Treatment adverse effects**: Patients' functional abilities and general health may be adversely affected by treatment. Patients may require routine laboratory tests to monitor medications.
- **Psychosocial needs**: Patients may become depressed and may lack transportation and financial resources. Patients may benefit from the assistance of a social worker, psychological therapy, and support groups.

Management of Clients with Disabilities

Elements of the case management of clients with disabilities include:

- Advocating for the disabled.
- Interviewing clients and reviewing healthcare records.
- Coordinating among healthcare providers.
- Assisting client to develop goals.
- Assessing client's needs and then continually reassessing.
- Developing a plan of care for appropriate interventions and modifying as needed.
- Contacting care providers and arranging for care/treatment/services.

Disability services are often provided by specialty units that focus on one type of disability, such as strokes, traumatic brain injury, or amputations. These units may consist of a team of staff in a center that serves many types of disabilities or in a separate facility. The case manager must determine the most appropriate rehabilitation program for the client and the accessibility. Some programs are centrally based, such as in a large city, and may not be readily available to clients outside of the area.

Alternative/Complementary Care Treatments

Case managers must be aware of all the healthcare options within their community in order to address the unique needs of a large, culturally diverse population. **Alternative or complementary care treatments** incorporate the concept of mind/body/spirit treatment, holistic medicine, and Eastern medicine. Some of these techniques may be administered within and combined with modern healthcare (e.g., massage during the childbirth process), some may be administered in alternative healthcare facilities (e.g., chiropractic care, acupuncture, and Reiki), and others are part of a growing alternative healthcare industry (e.g., guided imagery, dietary therapy, spiritual healing, herbal remedies, homeopathic treatments, tai chi, and yoga). There are also many treatment facilities for teenagers offering residential and experimental programs.

Adherence to Care Regimens

Adherence to care regimens on the part of the patient is essential if the target outcomes are to be achieved. Adherence is improved if patients actively participate in identifying problems and developing a plan of care. The case manager may utilize **motivational interviewing techniques** to engage the patient in the process. Adherence should be evidence-based, measurable, and linked directly to interventions. For example, for the problem of obesity with a goal of weight loss, an intervention could include maintaining a low-calorie diet and keeping a food diary. Measurement may involve monitoring the patient's weight. The case manager should maintain frequent contact with the patient and other care providers, discussing progress and identifying possible barriers to adherence before they become a problem. The case manager should provide the patient with information necessary for the patient to serve as his/her own advocate and to understand how the patient's actions may affect outcomes.

Problem and Opportunity Identification

The case manager should determine problems or opportunities that would be aided by case management interventions. This standard of practice involves multiple elements. Documentation of an agreement between the client, the client's support system or care provider, and the healthcare provider/organization that describes the identified problem or opportunity is necessary. Examples of opportunities for case management intervention may include the following: not having an evidence-based determined healthcare plan, not having established care plan goals, under- or overuse of healthcare services, utilization of numerous healthcare providers or healthcare services, and lack of appropriate support systems.

Individualized Treatment Plan

An individualized plan takes into account the support and resources within the client's family, friends, and community. The plan takes advantage of the client's resources in addressing the outstanding or immediate problems. The plan addresses all of the issues raised in the patient's assessment. The plan should include incremental steps toward improvement as well as expected outcomes. Use of formal agencies (e.g., mental health, Easter Seals) as well as folk support/community organizations (e.g., church grief support group, ESL tutoring, social organizations) available to assist with a particular issue are important to include in the plan. Development of good individualized plans requires the case manager have knowledge of and a relationship with people and places that welcome your clients and provide the experiences or support they need.

Quality Assurance Assessments

Clear **procedure and protocol manuals** must list the standards of care, list the quality assurance procedures, and be available to all staff. Client feedback should be sought in assessing the quality of the services provided. The following should be included in **quality assurance assessments**:

- Descriptions of communication tools (intake and follow up forms, partner notification, and risk-reduction counseling).
- Description of training provided to supervisors and staff along with job descriptions.
- Staff performance reviews.
- Chart reviews including initial assessment, prevention plan, and progress notes on clients.
- Presentation of cases by case managers to peers and supervisors that include intervention strategy discussions.
- Review by peers of the quality of services provided.
- Feedback from clients including satisfaction, concerns, and their ideas for improvements.
- Reviews and evaluations from outside professionals that verify that the promoted services are being delivered.

Medication Management Therapy and Reconciliation

Medication management therapy is a program that is administered by pharmacists. By involving pharmacists in such a program model, a patient garners enhanced understanding of his medical condition and the medication therapy that is required for the condition. It has been shown that having a pharmacist focus on a patient's medication therapy can decrease medication error risk, especially in the hospital setting, as pharmacists review and analyze interactions of different drugs that may be administered.

Medication reconciliation is an exhaustive process—the discharge medication list is reconciled with the admission medication list provided. This process can be quite effective in reducing medication errors and possible adverse drug reactions after a patient is discharged.

Medication Safety Assessment

Because the case manager has an overview of the client's medical conditions and treatments, often provided by multiple healthcare providers, the case manager should carry out a medication safety assessment:

- Assess achievement of treatment goals to determine if medications have been effective.
- Identify all medications, including OTC preparations, herbal preparations, and vitamins.
- Assess the client's actual use pattern for drugs, determining if the medications are taken as prescribed and are appropriate for the client's clinical needs.
- Determine the reason for the client failing to follow directions for medications, such as misunderstanding or inability to pay for medications.
- Identify duplications or medications that interact with each other.
- Identify all medication treatment problems, including the need for additional medications.
- Resolve medication issues with the assistance of physicians and collaboration of the client and/or caregivers. Social worker referral may be necessary if the client lacks the ability to pay for medications or, in some cases, less expensive medications may be substituted.
- Develop a new medication/treatment care plan in collaboration with client and/or caregivers.
- Carry out follow-up evaluations and reassess outcomes and achievement of therapeutic goals.

Physical Functioning and Behavioral Health Assessment

Importance of Client Assessment

The case manager has a responsibility to provide a comprehensive assessment of the patient's medical, intellectual, educational, psychological, social, religious, and financial status. Without an intimate understanding of the patient, a case manager's recommendations may lead to disastrous outcomes due to unrecognized barriers to care. The assessment is part of the patient's file and admissible in court if a suit is filed. Prepared assessment forms assist in gathering all needed information and should include, at a minimum, chief complaint; current diagnoses; current treatments including medications and the treatment plan; past medical history; social history including education level, family and community support system, sexual history and orientation, history of substance abuse, and religious affiliations and involvement; insurance eligibility; private and federal programs; the client's benefits package; and the expected outcomes of the case.

Standards of Client Assessment

Client assessment is a standard of practice in case management. The case manager performs a health assessment and a psychological assessment of each client. The case manager must be cognizant of any language barriers or cultural differences of the client in the scope of the assessments. The case manager should document the client's assessments using standardized criteria. The criteria need to be relative to the practice setting of the case manager. Examples of such criteria may include: physical/ functional ability, medical history, mental health history, intellectual ability, environmental setting, cultural/spiritual elements, or financial status.

Initial Client Assessment

The initial assessment must be a comprehensive and thorough attempt to develop an accurate profile of the client and the client's problem. The initial assessment may be done on an intake assessment form containing pre-established questions or may be the construction of a written narrative of their social history. In either case, it will cover the background of the current problem, current condition, living arrangements, relationships, and work experience. Part of the assessment must include the reason the client is seeking help as well as the initial or presenting problem. Discussion of the problem leads to what the client requires to bring stability and resolution. The client's personal strengths (e.g., education) and environment (e.g., family support) should be documented. Assessment of the client's ability to reason and understand options is a part of the assessment. The assessment is the foundation for the development of an individual plan for service or treatment.

Categories of Initial Assessment

The initial assessment covers the following **domains**:

Domain	Purpose of Assessment
Cognitive Function	Must be assessed to determine if the client can speak for themselves or if they need a proxy present to answer questions or participate in decision making
Diagnosis/Medical Conditions	Must be captured and a determination made of areas that may require the case manager's intervention
Medications	Can present potential problems with drug administration or interactions, and the case manager should arrange assistance if financial barriers exist
Care Access	Involves evaluating services for coordination of the services, obtaining providers or transportation, and negotiating costs
Functional Status	Covers activities of daily living (ADLs), instrumental activities of daily living (IADLs), and fall prevention
Social Situation	Evaluates the patient's support system and arranges social work intervention if needed
Nutritional Status	Impacts the overall health of the patient and the effectiveness of their medication
Emotional Status	The recognition of depression and other emotional disorders that can negatively impact the well-being of the patient, the care plan, and desired outcomes

Mental Status Exam

Case managers use observation in order to document a client's mental status. The client's situation, actions, speech, and appearance are taken into account in an abbreviated assessment (e.g., eminent hospitalization) or over an extended period of multiple interviews in order to document their mental status and capabilities in relationship to the services to be provided. It is important to always use a standardized form/questions in order to understand the client's emotional and cognitive processes. The **MSE** is not a separate, independent action, but is part of the overall intake process. Aside from general appearance, the case manager will note subtle visual and verbal clues about the client's thought process, impulse control, cognitive functioning and intelligence level, reality level and suicidal or homicidal tendencies. Active listening for both how and what the client says is important. Input from others is often necessary when the client either cannot provide information (e.g., about past events) or does not perform at an intellectual level in order to communicate for themselves (due to chronological age or from the effects of their disease).

Domains of a Functional Status Assessment

There are three domains or components of a functional status assessment:

1. **Activities of Daily Living** (ADL) include basic functions such as the ability to dress, bathe, feed, and toilet oneself. The level of independence is based in part on environmental factors: are stairs involved, is equipment needed to provide mobility, etc.
2. **Instrumental Activities of Daily Living** (IADLs) include the ability to do housework, shop, and prepare meals. Barriers in any of these areas may affect the ability to heal effectively or obtain/prepare food.
3. **Fall prevention** looks at the history of the patient as well as their future.

Review Video: Fall Prevention
Visit mometrix.com/academy and enter code: 972452

Identifying Acuity Levels

Patient classification systems and acuity tools are factors used to determine acuity or severity levels. These systems are utilized to determine appropriate staffing levels for healthcare services. When designing a patient classification system, the following elements must be considered: the physical layout or design of the facility, work shifts, vacations and holiday variances, and the policies and procedures of the organization. Some other elements to consider in the determination of acuity would be the skill of the staff, available technology, multidisciplinary support available, and existence of any clinical trials.

Magnuson Model

The Magnuson model is a model to determine the patient intensity or acuity level. This model represents the **acuity level** of the patient as well as the **complexity of the healthcare tasks** or services necessary to provide the required care to the patient. The acuity level or intensity level is the time requirement in the delivery of direct and indirect patient care. Acuity tools look at the patient intensity level and determine the hours of staffing time necessary. Such acuity tools enable both healthcare providers and administrators to analyze schedules and to determine the actual workload.

Roles and Functions of Case Managers and Other Providers

Role of Case Manager in Ergonomics

Ergonomics is the studying, designing, and arranging of safe and efficient interactions between people and things. Ergonomics has contributed to a healthy, productive, and safer work environment. Case managers have three (3) **areas for impact** on ergonomics in the workplace.

- The case manager may identify illnesses or injuries that occurred due to unsafe conditions on the job and report these to the appropriate company departments for further evaluation.
- When a job environment cannot be reasonably modified to accommodate a worker's limitations, the case manager may make referrals for strength or endurance training, work hardening, or vocational assessment or retraining.
- The case manager acts as an advocate for the worker, making the employer aware of the worker's limitations and working with the employer to modify the work environment, reduce work hours or responsibilities to allow lighter responsibilities during rehabilitation, or suggesting job-fit analysis to accommodate a permanently disabled worker.

Role of Case Manager in Patient Advocacy

In the role of the patient's advocate, the case manager is held to a "reasonable standard of care." This requires knowledge of what the **standard of care** is for the condition. This knowledge is obtained through education and up-to-date information on trends in medical, surgical and rehabilitation therapeutics. It is important for the case manager to understand the appropriateness of the procedure/provider to the patient's case. The case manager is not only responsible for their own actions in managing a case, but also the relationship between the patient and any vendors she recommends. Incidents that occur and are reported by either the vendor or the patient must be investigated with the findings documented and an action plan detailed.

Review Video: Patient Advocacy
Visit mometrix.com/academy and enter code: 202160

Role of Other Providers in Healthcare Management and Delivery

There may be a broad range of professional and nonprofessional providers in healthcare management and delivery. The roles of these other providers vary widely from limited patient contact to direct patient care and contact. The responsibilities of these other providers also vary considerably in the level of responsibility required. It is imperative that the roles and responsibilities of such providers be clearly and succinctly established. Examples of other providers in healthcare management and delivery may include mental health workers, health educators, community health workers, interpreters, nurses, medical assistants or licensed practical nurses, nutritionists, physicians, pharmacists, social workers, psychologists, and volunteers.

Role of the Payer's Claims Department in Case Management

There are many personnel involved in making claims payments and following the contract language in enforcing benefits. **Customer service representatives** are the first contact a person has for explanations of eligibility, coverage, and plan specifics. Claims are put into the payer system by a **claims processor**. Decisions on whether to approve, investigate, or deny claims is made by a **claims examiner**, usually the next job rung from a claims processor. **Claims supervisors** oversee the work flow of both processors and examiners and comprise the first level of management decision making. Final decisions regarding claims are usually the responsibility of the **claims manager**, although directors and vice presidents will be involved when unique situations arise or litigation might result. The **plan administrator** handles appeals, plan design and changes to a plan. If the plan is self-funded, one management-level person provides stop-loss advisories. **Case managers** may be involved in discussions between stop-loss carriers and the claims department liaison. The **account manager** handles service issues, complaints, and funding issues.

Role of Community Health Workers

Most of the roles and functions of other providers in healthcare management and delivery are self-explanatory. Community health workers serve to **facilitate the access** of patients to healthcare providers. These patients typically are the medically underserved in a community. Community health workers may also facilitate **technical and cultural links** between minority patients and healthcare providers in a community. Some examples of community health workers may include former drug addicts who educate IV drug users on the risks of HIV and hepatitis C, or cancer survivors who educate and advocate for cancer screening in at-risk patients. Typically, community health workers do not have licensure requirements or scope of practice laws.

Role of Community Vendors

Community vendors are those companies and organizations that provide supplies, equipment, and services to clients and healthcare organizations, such as hospitals, for a fee. Vendors may include various types of suppliers and contractors. Before doing business with a vendor, the case manager and/or health organization should always verify its legitimacy through a compliance officer, and the case manager should be aware that gifts to referral sources (such as the case manager or physician) from vendors may pose the risk of Stark Violations or Anti-Kickback statute violations. Community vendors that the case manager and clients do business with often include those that supply durable medical equipment, such as wheelchairs, walking aids (canes, walkers), commodes, and pressure pads and mattresses. Other vendors may provide hardware and software (encryption, electronic health records) used in healthcare as well as personal services, such as housecleaners and nurse aides.

Continuum of Care

Continuum of Care Model

The concept of the continuum of care is a model designed to manage a patient's or a certain population's medical problems. Currently, the continuum of care is a loosely organized system or chain in which healthcare-related services are not truly controlled as an integrated system. Ideally, the continuum of care model would enable a healthcare system to perform **audits** of its current system and services. Such audits would afford the healthcare system a means to identify strengths and weaknesses in their healthcare management system. This model can give a healthcare system a cross-sectional overview of efficient ways to integrate and avoid duplication of services.

Stages in the Continuum of Care

There are **five general stages in the continuum of care**:

1	General well-being and independence	This stage is one in which the patient is functionally independent and has good health with low health risk factors.
2	Predisposing risk factors and behaviors	At this stage, the patient has certain predisposing risks or behaviors for developing certain medical conditions.
3	Medical problem	At this juncture, a patient develops a medical problem that prompts him to action of some sort.
4	Treatment	At this point, a patient may opt to do nothing, self-treat, or undergo medical treatment.
5	Outcome	Depending upon the medical condition, the patient will return to good health, require continued treatment, or die.

Transitions of Care vs. Transitional Care

There is a distinction between transitions of care and transitional care.

- The American Geriatrics Society defines **transitional care** as the actions to assure the coordination and continuity of care as patients transfer between different locations or to different locations within the same facility. Locations may include hospitals, nursing homes, the patient's private home, physician's offices, and long-term care facilities. Transitional care involves logistics, patient education, and the cooperation of the various healthcare providers involved.
- **Transitions of care** refers to the movement of patients between locations, healthcare providers, or different levels of care within the same facility as the healthcare needs or healthcare condition of the patient changes. Transitions of care is a narrower subset of the broader concept of transitional care.

PITFALLS IN TRANSITIONS OF CARE

Often, patient care for a serious illness can require multiple settings (both acute and long-term care) and the involvement of numerous healthcare providers. The one essential and fundamental basic in transitions of care is that of **communication** between all involved. Some of the pitfalls in the transitions of care and miscommunication can include patient/care-provider confusion as to the medical condition involved and the care needed, absence of referral follow-up, medication errors, inadequate or spotty patient monitoring, and the increase in cost due to duplication of healthcare services.

NATIONAL TRANSITIONS OF CARE COALITION

The National Transitions of Care Coalition has helped to identify certain types of patients who are quite vulnerable to the pitfalls in transitions of care. Some of these patients include patients that do not speak English, patients of a different cultural background, children with special healthcare needs, the frail elderly, persons with cognitive impairments, persons with complex medical conditions, adults with disabilities, people at the end of life, low-income patients, patients who move frequently such as retirees and those with unstable health insurance coverage, and behavioral healthcare patients.

Chapter Quiz

Ready to see how well you retained what you just read? Scan the QR code to go directly to the chapter quiz interface for this study guide. If you're using a computer, simply visit the bonus page at **mometrix.com/bonus948/ccm** and click the Chapter Quizzes link.

Reimbursement Methods

Transform passive reading into active learning! After immersing yourself in this chapter, put your comprehension to the test by taking a quiz. The insights you gained will stay with you longer this way. Scan the QR code to go directly to the chapter quiz interface for this study guide. If you're using a computer, simply visit the bonus page at **mometrix.com/bonus948/ccm** and click the Chapter Quizzes link.

Insurance Principles

Major Types of Health Insurance Coverage

Major types of health insurance coverage include the following:

- **Indemnity health insurance plan** is a legal entity, licensed by the state insurance department, providing reimbursement for healthcare claims. Managed indemnity companies are those who have adopted cost-saving approaches to healthcare coverage.
- **Self-insured** is an alternative option adopted by many companies where all or part of the coverage risk, up to a threshold amount, is assumed by the employer rather than an insurance company. For costs incurred over the individual employee's threshold amount, the employer purchases a re-insurance or stop-loss policy, which then pays the remainder of a claim.
- **Automobile insurance** provides coverage for medical expenses and lost wages when the car owner/policy holder has an accident. They must also be aware that when auto insurance maximums are reached, the healthcare plan may be used to complete treatment. Many auto accident cases go to court and the case management records may be subpoenaed.
- **Managed care** is a cost-containment healthcare system overseen by an organization other than the physician or patient. Managed care encompasses HMOs (health maintenance organizations), PPOs (preferred provider organizations), EPOs (exclusive provider organizations), and POS (point of service) plans.

Insurance Coverage Concepts

Key concepts when discussing insurance coverage include the following:

- Insurance plans or issuers can require a waiting period before the start of coverage. **Preexisting conditions waiting period** begins when the policy waiting period begins, not the first day of insurance coverage.
- **Creditable coverage** references the time during which a person is covered by health insurance, including COBRA continuation coverage.
- A significant **break in coverage** is a span of 63 days or more without health insurance. To calculate creditable coverage, credit is granted to coverage without any break in that coverage of 63 days or more. Coverage that ended more than 63 days from the new enrollment will not be credited against a **preexisting condition**. A certificate of coverage must be issued by group health plans and health insurance issuers.

Key Considerations in Insurance Coverage

Key considerations in insurance coverage include the following:

- **Hospital length of stay** is defined as the duration of an inpatient hospital stay, calculated in days. Length of stay for newborns begins at the time of the newborn's delivery or the last delivery time in the event of multiple births when the birth occurs at a hospital. If the delivery occurs outside the hospital, length of stay begins at the time the mother or newborn is admitted to the hospital in connection with the childbirth. Only the physician can determine that the admittance is "in connection with childbirth."
- **Ancillary services** are those diagnostic and therapeutic services needed by a patient other than nursing or medicine. These include respiratory, laboratory, radiology, nutrition, physical and occupational therapy, and pastoral services.
- **Interventions** are the planned strategies and activities that address a maladaptive behavior or state of being and assist growth and change. Another term for intervention is treatment when used to describe medical treatment strategies. Examples of interventions are advocacy, psychotherapy, or speech language therapy.

Long-Term Care Cases

A payers' **relationship** with the case manager is important for smooth implementation of long-term cases. **Honesty** with the payer is very important, including communication of patient setbacks. The level of involvement of a case manager is dependent on the patient's medical history, age, diagnosis, current medical situation, treatment plan and required services, family and community support, timing of receiving the case, and the patient's benefit plan. One major benefit of case management is the early identification of a possible long-term case to document services needed and implement cost controls. Other benefits of long-term care case management include cost containment, the creation of a case presentation of findings to the referral source, improvements in the patient's situation due to case management, the presence of an attainable objective that can help maintain an encouraging attitude with the patient and family, and the identification of an end goal that reflects the patient's wishes. Cases of terminal illness are more stressful on the patient and family, and can benefit from opportunities to clarify direction and ensure that the patient's comfort and end-of-life wishes are emphasized in the long-term care plan. This may provide comfort to the patient and family amidst a situation that is otherwise out of their control.

Challenges

Long-term care is characterized by long periods of slow, insignificant progress or plateaus as well as the hurdles of dealing with changing providers and possibly case managers. Changes in providers causes stress for both the patient and their family and can cause a temporary setback. Case managers need to reestablish their relationship with the new providers to provide patient information. Long-term cases often incur **complications**, including short-term illness, degradation of the primary condition or introduction of new diagnoses that change the treatment plan. Changing family or home care situations also impact the treatment plan. Aging parents may indicate the need for transfer of patient services from the home to a facility. The financial burden of a long-term illness requires review of the patient and/or family's finances on a regular basis.

Health Policy Reimbursement

Private health insurance may cover the cost of long-term care when medically necessary. If the limit of private insurance is reached or care is considered custodial, **Medicaid** may cover the costs.

Medicare, however, does not cover the cost of long-term care. Medicare covers short-term care in a skilled nursing facility (SNF), provided the care is required following a qualified hospital stay.

- Medicare pays 100% of the first 20 days in a SNF.
- For days 21-100, the patient pays $209.50 per day (as of 2025) and then Medicare pays any balance past that.
- After day 100, the patient is responsible for the full cost of the SNF.

Skilled nursing and sub-acute care placements require the case manager to understand specific policy benefits and whether or not the insurer will coordinate payment with Medicare. Most insurers make very little distinction between intermediate and custodial care in distributing benefits. Inpatient rehabilitation has specific qualifiers for private policies that may or may not be the same as the Medicare admission criteria.

Financial Burden

Long-term cases place a financial burden on the families and the payers. It is important for case managers to make sure these cases are not prematurely closed. Long-term cases provide a situation requiring smart negotiation skills by the case manager. A long-term case guarantees income to the providers and presents an opportunity for the case manager to negotiate a reduced rate for a long-term contract. Conversely, once an established case becomes long-term or the need for services change, the case manager should renegotiate the vendor's rate to benefit the payer and the family. (This **cost-containment measure** is important to capture in the case manager's report.) To assist families in dealing with the financial burden of long-term case care, the case manager may need to supply information on **alternative funding sources** (public or private) and assist with applications for aide.

Red Flags for Payers

A red flag is an indication that the case is not routine and will usually benefit from the services of a case manager. Different types of insurance require different definitions of red flags. Workers' compensation claims often use lost-time at work guidelines for red flags. Catastrophic illnesses are red flags for group medical insurance plans, as are premature births or chronic and devastating long-term illnesses. Multiple hospitalizations and multiple physicians are a red flag indicator that extenuating circumstances, beyond the admitting diagnosis, are in existence and may benefit from case management. The types of services ordered are also a red flag indicator of cases that may benefit from case management. Case managers work with insurance claims departments to uncover potentially serious cases. Curiosity, instinct, and a paper trail are the clues to streamlining medical care and cost containment measures.

Red Flags for Long-Term Case Management

Long-term case management is usually determined by the **diagnosis** (e.g., multiple sclerosis, spinal cord injury, amputation, elderly end-of-life) and **prognosis** for cases requiring services for several months, years, or a lifetime. Red flags must be recognized and case management intervention initiated when an illness or treatment has a potential for long term treatment. Examples of common **red flags for long term care** needs include the following:

- Lack of improvement, setbacks, or complications in routine cases.
- Terminal illness.
- Whenever treatment is 6 months or longer.
- Presence of multiple medical conditions.
- An increase in complications, which is an indicator of possible systemic issues.

Workers' Compensation

Workers' compensation provides coverage of injury or illness that occurs while an individual was at work or that was caused by a work-related task. The premiums are paid by the employer and the initial intent of the legislation was as an incentive for employers to increase workers' safety. Some benefits vary by state, however, payment of medical bills related to illness, injury, or occupational diseases (e.g., black lung) as well as a percentage of lost wages is provided by workers' compensation. There are also benefits in case of death and total or partial disability of the employee. If a worker is covered by and accepts coverage under workers' compensation, they may not claim benefits under a group insurance policy or bring suit against the employer for work-related injuries. It is very important for case managers to have documentation in the individual's plan if the case is being handled through workers' compensation.

Role of Case Management

Returning an employee to work is the goal of case management in workers' compensation claims. Early case management facilitates proper and timely medical care, creates good public relations with employees, reduces the cost of health care, and aggressive case management reduces lost work time. Case manager communication with providers facilitates a return to light-duty work, an adjustment in work requirements, or a change in atmosphere allowing return to work. An overview of medical care provided by multiple sources prevents duplication of services. A case manager can assist in obtaining the highest quality of care as well as negotiating discounts and assisting in containment of costs through appropriate physician selection. A case manager facilitates communication between all involved parties: employer, insurance adjustor, providers, employee, and family.

Reimbursement and Payment Methodologies

Primary Financial Resource Methods in Reimbursement

There are five primary financial resource methods in **healthcare reimbursement**. One such method is **state, county, and municipality taxes**. Taxes at such levels of government serve to fund various models of healthcare reimbursement. In universal healthcare systems in other countries, most of the funding is obtained through general taxation. In numerous countries with universal health care, certain **levies** are also assessed to supplement general taxation revenues for healthcare reimbursement. Social health insurance, private/voluntary health insurance, out-of-pocket payment, and donations also serve as financial resources in healthcare reimbursement. Most healthcare systems utilize a mixture of all five methods.

Rules for Reimbursement

An integral component of prospective payment systems is **diagnosis-related groups (DRGs)**. DRGs essentially categorize medical and surgical services in groups related to a diagnosis. Services needed to treat patients are "**bundled**," and reimbursement rates cover routine patient care costs. The reimbursement rate is based on the average cost of care for a patient with a particular diagnosis. Services delivered by medical providers are reimbursed by procedure codes according to the Physician Medicare Fee Schedule. Acute care facilities are reimbursed at the predetermined rate that Medicare pays for inpatient services under the PPS plan. Skilled nursing facilities are paid by the total reimbursable per diem Medicaid rate established by the facility's comptroller.

Reimbursement Methods

Case rate reimbursement: A specific reimbursement is paid based on an agreement reached between the payer and the healthcare providers. This payment covers the costs of a specific group of treatments and services, such as obstetric services and surgical services. For example, a managed care program may contract to pay a specific fee for CABG.

Bundled reimbursement: Care is reimbursed according to expected costs for a clinical episode of care: for example, a bundled payment may include the costs for hospitalization and physician care. CMS has developed the Bundled Payments for Care Improvement (BPCI) initiative and is testing 4 models of reimbursement:

- CMS pays for inpatient episode of care with physicians paid separately.
- CMS pays for inpatient episode, post-acute care, and service for 90 days based on a retrospective system, where actual expenditures are considered along with target expenditures, and then reimbursement is either increased or recouped.
- Similar to model 2 but begins with post-acute care.
- CMS pays a prospectively-determined rate for an episode of care that covers all hospital and physician services.

Prospective Payment Systems

Prospective payment systems (PPSs) are designed to encourage healthcare providers to deliver efficient and effective patient care without overusing services. This concept originally began with health maintenance organizations (HMOs). HMOs get a flat monthly premium and are to provide any services that a patient may need. This system has inherent incentives for healthcare providers to manage patients and their treatment in an efficient and cost-effective manner. Medicare prospective payment systems for hospitals, skilled nursing facilities, and home healthcare agencies are quite similar to the HMO model. With Medicare PPS, the facility gets a single payment to cover a defined time period or inpatient stay as opposed to a monthly premium. The payment is based upon diagnoses and standard functional assessments.

Determining Medical Necessity for Reimbursement

Insurance companies have **Medical Directors** (state licensed physicians) who oversee claims and determine benefit eligibility for treatment/procedures. The following are procedures followed to document whether or not the facts of the case present a medical necessity. Foremost, policies must clearly state that **medical necessity** must be shown for procedures/treatments. Subscribers must have a clear expectation of coverage. If benefits are denied, this is done only following review by the medical director. Denials should never be based on a monetary incentive. Cases involving high risk procedures (e.g., transplants) or infants in intensive care or oncology wards should have closer review by the medical director, risk manager and possibly corporate counsel. Medical directors should seek guidance from specialists for cases that are outside their area of expertise. To gain a complete clinical picture, medical directors should speak with the attending physician. Medical directors must carefully document their reviews of medical records, including time and date of the review of each piece of information. The company should maintain a database of denials in order to assure consistency. Additionally, a regular review of legal cases will assist in avoiding unwarranted denials.

Coordination of Benefits

When someone has more than one health insurance plan, coordination of payments must be done so that no more than 100% of the cost of medical care is reimbursed. Any insurance plan that does not contain **COB provisions** must pay for medical care first to avoid overpayment of fees. The following rules apply to COB:

1. Employee insurance plans pay first.
2. A plan that covers the individual as a dependent pays second.
3. If a dependent is covered by multiple plans, the plan of the employee with the first birth date pays first, but only if both plans use the birthday rule and the parents are married.
4. If the plans do not use the birthday rule and the parents are married, the male parent's plan pays first.
5. If the parents are divorced, the court-appointed primary responsible parent's plan pays first.
6. If parents are divorced and there is no court-determined primary responsible parent, then the plan of the custodial parent pays first, followed by the plan of the spouse of the custodial parent, followed by the plan of the parent without custody, and finally the plan of the spouse of the parent without custody.
7. Active employee plans pay before inactive (retired) employee plans.
8. Plans covering an individual as an employee or a dependent pay before a COBRA plan.
9. If none of the preceding rules provide determination of the order of payment, then the plan in place for the longest time pays first.

Health Care Delivery Systems

In the United States, healthcare delivery systems are traditionally fragmented, unique, and quite complex in nature. In contrast to the United States, most other countries in developed nations have national health insurance systems, which are commonly referred to as **universal access systems**. Such universal access systems are managed by the government and are funded by taxes. Healthcare delivery systems in the United States consist of subcategories such as managed care, military, vulnerable populations, and integrated service delivery. **Managed care healthcare delivery systems** are the predominant systems for the delivery of health care in the United States.

Managed Care Healthcare Delivery System

The managed care healthcare delivery system promotes efficiency by the integration of basic functions of healthcare delivery and uses management strategies to control healthcare service usage. Managed healthcare delivery systems also determine the **prices** of services and provider reimbursement. The government and employers primarily provide the financing for managed care systems. Managed care delivery systems act like insurance companies in that they use a contract health plan that is an agreement between the managed care system and the subscriber. Subscribers under a managed care delivery system are usually required to use selected healthcare providers.

ACCOUNTABLE CARE ORGANIZATIONS

Accountable care organizations (ACOs), established per the *Affordable Care Act*, are groups of physicians, hospitals, and other healthcare providers who voluntarily establish partnerships or agreements to provide care to Medicare patients. The purpose of ACOs is to improve delivery of quality care while saving healthcare costs. ACOs avoid duplication of services through coordination of care. Medicare shares healthcare savings generated to participating providers. The different types of ACOs include:

- **Shared savings program**: Payment is made for participants under fee-for-service who meet performance standards while lowering costs.
- **Advance payment model:** This is a supplementary program to the shared savings program. Participants receive monthly upfront payments to invest in staff and infrastructure needs to better meet goals.
- **Pioneer model:** Original model available to those who had already established groups. Shared savings and payments were generally higher than in current plans. No longer accepting applicants.

Private Benefit Programs

HMOs

The **four models** of HMOs include the following:

- **Staff model** is comprised of physicians who work only for, and are paid by the HMO and who see only the HMO's patients.
- **Group model** is characterized by a group of physicians who contract with the HMO to provide services for a fixed monthly rate per enrollee (capitated rate), but are not HMO employees.
- **Independent Practice Association (IPA) model** is a legal entity sponsored by physicians that contracts with HMOs and are bound by the terms of that contract. The physicians have their own practice and see their own patients as well as care for the HMO's enrollees at the HMO contract rate. The IPA negotiates with the HMO for payment by a capitated fee or a discounted, fee-for-service rate.
- **Network model** is one in which the HMO contracts directly with IPAs, medical groups, and independent physicians forming a provider network. Provider payments are by a capitated fee or a discounted, fee-for-service rate.

GATEKEEPER, PPO, EPO, AND POS

A **Gatekeeper** is a primary care physician who oversees, authorizes, and coordinates patient medical care that is outside their own practice. Healthcare beyond the gatekeeper must be approved in order to be reimbursed. Gatekeepers are a cost control mechanism as well as means of directing patients to in-network providers. True medical or surgical emergencies and routine gynecological care are exempt from gatekeeper referrals.

Preferred provider organizations (PPO) are a large group of medical providers providing medical services on a negotiated or discounted fee-for-service schedule. Enrollees pay a higher coinsurance if they receive services outside the PPO.

Exclusive provider organizations (EPO) use a network of contracted physicians who care for enrollees at a discounted rate. Enrollees are not reimbursed for care received from a provider not part of the EPO.

Point of Service (POS) plans are a combination of PPO and HMO plans using a contracted network of providers and a primary care physician as gatekeeper to control specialty referrals. Reimbursements for care that is provided by out-of-network physicians are subject to higher deductibles and coinsurance amounts.

Employer-Sponsored Health Coverage

Typically, an employer offering an employer-sponsored health insurance benefit has to make a large payment contribution towards the cost of the insurance coverage. On average, employers pay about 85% of the premium for the employee and 75% of the premium for the employee's dependents. The employee pays the remainder of the premium, and it is usually paid through pretax earnings. Many smaller employers don't have the financial ability to offer employer-sponsored health coverage. For those that do, insurance coverage options are similar to those offered to large firms. Some small employers choose self-funded healthcare plans in which the company utilizes its own capital/funds to offer health benefits to employees as opposed to paying an insurance company.

Third-Party Administrators

A third-party administrator (TPA) performs administrative functions for self-insured employers. The services include, but are not limited to, performing claims review and payment, maintaining records, reporting on utilization, providing case management, and overseeing the provider network. Using a TPA usually provides significant costs savings over the company administering its self-insurance internally. A TPA decreases the startup time by providing computerization of the healthcare plan and administrative expertise. A TPA eliminates the expense of hiring employees to oversee the insurance program. TPA fees cover the computer costs involved in maintaining the self-insurance and meeting all **HIPAA requirements**. A TPA also provides objectivity in claims review as they are not direct employees of the company. Furthermore, a TPA provides consulting services to the company on state and federal regulations regarding insurance plans, since self-insurance avoids minimum benefits required by state and federal regulations.

Individually Purchased Health Insurance

Approximately 7% of Americans purchase individual health insurance, according to the US Census Bureau. Individuals have a comparable menu of products to those rendered by employer-sponsored programs. Major medical insurance is usually purchased by an individual and results in increased out-of-pocket costs in the form of higher deductibles and higher copayments. The person pays the whole premium, and most do not receive any tax benefits; however, self-employed individuals may receive a tax deduction. Individually purchased health insurance is mainly regulated at the state level, and premiums can vary greatly depending upon age and health status.

Pharmacy Benefits Management

Pharmacy benefits management (PBM) involves companies that give prescription drug benefit programs to employers and to health insurance carriers. PBMs contract with various entities and provide managed drug benefits. PBMs may contract with managed care organizations; self-insured employers; health insurance companies; Medicaid; Medicare; unions; and local, state, and federal government entities. Tools that PBMs use to manage prescription drug benefits include price, utilization, drug mix, and combination (formularies and disease management programs).

Home Care Coverage

Private insurance plans usually will cover some of the costs of home care on an acute basis; however, long-term service benefits may vary among different plans. They usually pay for skilled professional care services with the provision of cost sharing. Few private insurers may pay for personal care services. Most private insurers will pay for comprehensive hospice care. Some people have to buy Medigap coverage or purchase long-term care insurance to meet home care needs. Long-term care insurance originally protected individuals from huge costs that come with a prolonged nursing home stay. Currently, some long-term care insurers have increased coverage to include some in-home services.

COBRA

If a patient was formerly employed and health insurance was provided by the employer or by a union, a federal law known as COBRA provides a guarantee of continued health coverage for a period of time after leaving that employment. **COBRA** is extremely important for a patient with a pre-existing health condition. **High-deductible** insurance policies are another option for uninsured or underinsured patients. **Short-term** insurance coverage may be a viable option for the uninsured if they are not pregnant and generally in good health; it is usually a temporary form of health insurance that may last from one month to one year. High-risk insurance pools, state-sponsored health insurance for children, Medicaid, the Bureau of Primary Care, state health departments, and prescription assistance programs are also resources for the uninsured and the underinsured.

Employer-Based Wellness Programs

Employer-based health and wellness programs are those programs provided by the employer to benefit the health of the employees and include:

- **Health risk assessment**: May include screening, such as for high blood pressure and diabetes, as well as routine physical examinations.
- **Weight loss and fitness programs**: May include slowing elevators to encourage people to use the stairs, stocking cafeterias and vending machines with healthy foods, carrying out weight loss contests, encouraging participation in exercise programs, and establishing support groups.
- **Smoking cessation programs**: These programs provide education and support to those willing to quit smoking and may be coupled with financial incentives. Most smoking cessation programs last for at least 4 weeks.
- **Employee assistance programs**: Part of the benefit package offered employees in many organizations to assist employees with personal or work-related problems that interfere with their ability to carry out their jobs. While EAPs vary, they usually include counseling services and referrals.

Public Benefit Programs

CHIP and OASDI

CHIP is the joint state and federal **Children's Health Insurance Program**. It was established in 1997 by the federal government to provide matching funds to states for health insurance coverage for children. States set their eligibility following federal guidelines. Recipients must be under the age of 19, have low income (determined by the state's income range), be determined as ineligible for Medicaid, and can have no other health insurance coverage. CHIP covers, at a minimum, inpatient and outpatient hospital services; doctors' surgical and medical services; laboratory and x-ray services; and well-baby/child care, including immunizations.

OASDI is the **Old-Age, Survivors, and Disability Insurance** program which is the centerpiece of the Social Security Act. It provides hospital insurance to the elderly and supplementary medical insurance for other medical costs.

Social Security Disability Insurance

Social Security Disability Insurance (SSDI) is overseen by the Social Security Administration. It is a federal program of the United States government and is funded by payroll taxes. SSDI is utilized to provide supplemental income to people who have employment restrictions due to disability. SSDI may be temporary or permanent and is based upon the status of the disability. SSDI does not depend upon the person's income. According to the Social Security Administration, SSDI qualifications include a physical/mental condition preventing substantial gain activity, the expected length of condition is 12 months or death, age less than 65, and is available when 20 Social Security credits have been accumulated in the 10 years prior to disability.

Supplemental Security Income

Supplemental Security Income (SSI) is a federal program run by the Social Security Administration, but using general tax funds to provide supplemental income to the aged or any age person who is blind or disabled. To receive SSI, the individual does not need to be receiving Social Security benefits, but must have very **limited income and personal property**. Limited income is federally defined as monthly income less than $967 for an individual and less than $1,450 for a couple (2025). Limited personal property is federally defined as less than $2000 in assets for an individual and less than $3000 for a couple (2025). Individual states may have slightly different definitions and requirements. Not all income and property are considered when determining eligibility. For instance, most housing and food assistance is excluded, as are assets such as a home, a car, wedding rings, business property, and reasonable allowances for household items and burial expenses.

SSI Eligibility under disability applies to any individual, regardless of age, who cannot engage in substantial gainful employment, cannot work due to a medically diagnosed physical or mental impairment, or whose medical impairment will result in death or in a disability lasting 12 months or more. SSI payments are independent of any Social Security benefits. Most SSI recipients also receive medical care paid for through the Medicaid program. The base monthly SSI payment is $967 for an individual or $1,450 for a couple (2025), minus any income that is considered, but most states further supplement SSI.

Centers for Medicare and Medicaid Services

The Centers for Medicare and Medicaid Services (CMS) is a federal agency that runs the Medicare and Medicaid programs providing benefits to over 75 million Americans. It also covers the Children's Health Insurance Program (CHIP). CMS also has responsibility to regulate laboratory testing on humans (except research) and, along with the departments of Labor and Treasury, assists in maintaining health insurance coverage for small companies and individuals and eliminating discrimination based on health status for people purchasing health insurance. CMS combats fraud and abuse in cooperation with federal departments and state and local governments. CMS helps improve the quality of healthcare for people receiving health coverage via its programs through development and enforcement of standards, measuring and improving outcomes of care, and educating healthcare providers and beneficiaries.

Review Video: Medicare & Medicaid
Visit mometrix.com/academy and enter code: 507454

MEDICARE

Medicare is a federally directed program that was introduced by the Title XIX Social Security Act in 1965. It is the nation's largest health insurance program covering over 40 million Americans. It provides health insurance to elderly patients and to patients with disabilities. The patient who is covered will receive hospital, doctor, and further medical care as needed. The patient's income is not a factor for eligibility. Original Medicare consists of Part A and Part B, and covers the majority of medical care when the patient seeks care at a facility that accepts Medicare. If the patient requires prescription drug assistance, they may opt into Part D, which is the Medicare drug plan, or they may opt into the Medicare Advantage Plan (Part C), which bundles Parts A, B and D.

Medicare covers people who are:

- **65 years old** and receiving or eligible for benefits through the Social Security or Railroad Retirement systems or if the patient's spouse has Medicare-covered government employment.
- **Disabled**, but only once they are on Social Security disability benefits for 24 months and have completed the five-month waiting period; i.e., a total of 29 months.
- **Diagnosed with permanent kidney failure or end-stage renal disease** (ESRD), meaning they are on dialysis or require a transplant. Social Security or Railroad retirement benefits must also be met and they have a 3-month waiting period before benefits begin. Benefits end 3 months following the end of dialysis or 36 months following a transplant. Illness other than ESRD is not covered for people who do not meet regular Medicare eligibility. If a patient is already enrolled in a Medicare Managed Care Plan/Health Maintenance Organization (HMO), the plan will cover their kidney failure treatments; otherwise they cannot join a plan once diagnosed.

MEDICARE PART A

Medicare Part A covers hospital care (inpatient), care at a skilled nursing facility or nursing home, hospice care, and home health care. Hospital treatment payment with traditional Medicare Part A is as follows:

- In-hospital days 1 to 60
  - Medicare pays 100% of allowable charges minus deductible
  - Patient pays Part A deductible = $1,676 (for 2025)
- In-hospital days 61 to 90
  - Medicare pays 100% of allowable charges minus Part A coinsurance
  - Patient pays Part A coinsurance = $419/day (for 2025)

Reimbursement Methods

- In-hospital days 91 and beyond
    - Medicare pays for 60 lifetime reserve days. Once these are used, all costs accrued after 90 days of hospitalization are 100% the responsibility of the patient.
    - Patient cost when using lifetime reserve days = $838/day (for 2025)

Each time the patient is out of the hospital for 60 days they begin a new benefit period if admitted again and must pay their deductible again, even if admission is in the same year.

Medicare Part B

Medicare Part B covers both medically necessary services and preventive services such as doctor visits, physical therapy, occupational therapy, speech therapy, medical equipment, assessments, clinical research, mental health support and wellness visits. The patient has to **pay a monthly premium for Medicare Part B,** which is either directly billed to the patient or deducted from their Social Security or other benefit payment. This premium is based on the patient's income. The program covers 80% of the authorized expense for any medical attention that is required (following a yearly deductible).

Medigap and Medicare Select

Patients are responsible for Medicare's coinsurance, deductible fees and many medical services not covered, e.g., prescriptions. **Medigap** is private insurance that helps pay these "gaps." Medigap's open enrollment period is 6 months from the date of enrollment in Medicare Part B and age 65 or older. Open enrollment means the patient cannot be turned down or charged higher premiums due to poor health, factors that limit Medigap options after the open enrollment period.

Another type of supplemental health insurance is Medicare Select. **Medicare Select** is a health maintenance organization-type policy that specifies the hospitals and in some cases the providers a patient must use, unless there is an emergency. Due to the provider restrictions, Medicare Select usually offers more reasonable premiums than Medigap policies.

Indications that Private Policy Will pay First

Many people have both Medicare and private health insurance coverage. The **private policy will pay first** in any of the following cases:

- The patient is 65 or older, and the patient or spouse works for a company (20 or more employees) that provides a group health plan.
- The patient is disabled, and the patient or family member works for a company (100 or more employees) that provides a large group health plan.
- The patient has End-Stage Renal Disease and either group plan coverage or COBRA, and is within his or her first 30 months of Medicare eligibility.
- The patient is covered for the illness or injury under workers' compensation, the federal black lung program, or no-fault or liability insurance.

DURABLE MEDICAL EQUIPMENT

Durable medical equipment (DME) is equipment that generally can only be used for medical purposes, is durable (as opposed to disposable, although some items, such as colostomy supplies, are actually disposable), and is used in the home environment. DME includes a wide variety of items, such as commode chairs, hospital beds, walker, wheelchairs, CPAP machines, infusion pumps, blood sugar monitors and supplies, and suction equipment. DME is covered (80%) by Medicare B, but coverage requires that both the ordering physician and the supplier be enrolled in Medicare, and those suppliers who do not accept Medicare assignment are not limited in how much they can charge. Medicare is currently phasing in a competitive bidding program for suppliers of DME for those enrolled in original Medicare (not Medicare Advantage) in order to cut costs, and this can change the suppliers and Medicare payments. Private insurance policies usually cover all or part of the costs of durable medical equipment, but this may vary.

CASE MANAGER'S ROLE IN OBTAINING DME

Durablé medical equipment must be appropriate for use in the home, have a medical/therapeutic purpose, withstand repeated use, allow sterilization or disinfection between uses, and not be useful in the absence of illness or injury. Durable medical equipment may be

- A **basic mobility device** such as a walker or crutches.
- An **assistive device** for activities of daily living such as bathroom equipment and incontinence, wound care, or feeding/kitchen aids.
- **Extensive mobility equipment** such as a wheelchair, motorized scooter, or hospital bed.
- **Advanced high-tech equipment** such as oxygen, ventilator, infusion pump, or sleep monitor.

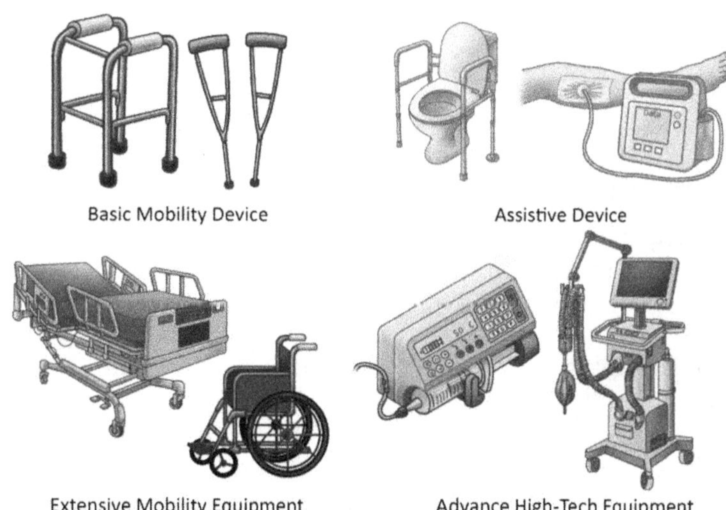

Case managers must understand the equipment handled by various vendors and establish a relationship with the vendors in order to offer the patient a choice of vendors and monitor/report on the success of the patient. The vendor assists the case manager by procuring equipment at the appropriate time, setting up the equipment, instructing the patient and their caregivers on the use of the equipment, handling repairs/replacement of equipment, and completing insurance paperwork.

Case Manager's Role in Monitoring DME

The case manager has the responsibility to monitor a patient's use of durable medical equipment, amend their **individualized treatment plan** as changes in the need for use of the equipment occur, and report on the overall relationship with the vendor. Vendors should assist or at least supply criteria for the proposed equipment. In ordering and placing equipment in the home, the case manager must be aware of the physical layout of the house so that equipment that cannot be operated in the space available will not be ordered. The physical dimensions of the patient must be taken into account as well as changes that will occur over the duration of the equipment use (e.g., children's growth, reduction in weight, small adults needing child-size equipment). The case manager must determine if the patient is using the equipment correctly or not at all, removing unused equipment. **Progressive disabilities** need close monitoring to adjust equipment in accordance with the advance of the disease. For long term disabilities, it may be more economical to purchase versus rent equipment. Case managers can work with vendors to arrange for rental fees to be applied to purchases, documenting the information for presentation to the insurance provider.

Medicaid

Medicaid is a national insurance program, created by **Title XIX** of the Social Security Act, for the poor and "needy" in all states and territories. There are no out-of-pocket medical expenses for persons covered by Medicaid. Medicaid is funded by federal and state governments and usually administered by state welfare or health departments. Although coverage varies from state to state/territory, it must always cover the following:

- Inpatient hospital care and outpatient services.
- Physician services.
- Skilled nursing homes for adults.
- Laboratory and x-ray services.
- Family planning services.
- Preventative and periodic screening, diagnosis, and treatment for children under age 21.

Categorically Needy and Medically Needy

Title XIX of the Social Security Act established Medicaid as a national insurance program for the poor and categorically or medically needy. States set the eligibility requirements using the minimum standards set by CMS.

- **Categorically needy** are families and certain children who qualify for public assistance, e.g., Temporary Assistance for Needy Families (TANF) or Supplemental Security Income (SSI), and include the aged, blind, and physically disabled adults and children.
- **Medically needy** are eligible individuals or families with sufficient earnings to meet their basic needs but do not have the resources to pay healthcare bills. Low income is not the only criteria for Medicaid eligibility; assets and other resources are considered. Medically needy often qualify for coverage due to excessive medical expenses and the benefits may be confined to that specific illness only, e.g., tuberculosis (TB).

Qualifications for Categorically Needy

Various individuals/groups must receive Medicaid categorically needy assistance:

- Patients deemed categorically needy by their state, and receive financial support from various federal assistance programs.
- Individuals receiving Federal Supplemental Security income (SSI).
- Patients that are older than 65 that are blind or have complete disability.
- Pregnant women and children younger than 6 years of age who live in families that are up to 133% of the federal poverty level (some states allow for a higher income to meet eligibility in this class).
- Adults under the age of 65 that make less than or equal to 133% of the federal poverty level and are not receiving Medicare.
- Families who receive adoption assistance and foster care under Title IV-E of the Social Security Act.

Guidelines for Categorically Needy

Medicaid funds are provided to states that apply more liberal guidelines for categorically needy families, such as:

- Infants up to age 1 and pregnant women whose income is below 185% of the federal poverty level (or the percentage set by the state) and not covered under the mandatory rules.
- Some aged, blind, or disabled adults whose income is above the mandatory coverage limit but below the federal poverty level.
- Certain women needing breast or cervical cancer treatment.
- Institutionalized individuals with income and resources below specified limits.
- Individuals receiving care via home and community-based services but who would be eligible if institutionalized.
- Individuals receiving hospice care.
- TB-infected individuals who meet the financial eligibility for Medicaid at the SSI level for their TB-related ambulatory services and TB drugs only.

Coordination with Social Programs

Many recipients of Medicaid are underinsured, economically disadvantaged, and coping with life problems that are not related to their illness. This population contains the elderly as well as families who are unemployed or underemployed. The biggest challenge is keeping the patients enrolled in a plan that can provide coordinated services. Finding health providers who will accept Medicaid is one problem, however, basic human needs are often the most pressing problems: obtaining food, housing, clothing, and transportation. Case managers must be able to identify clinical as well as social needs and **work in tandem with social workers** when applicable. Arranging meals-on-wheels or homemaker assistance for the elderly, coordinating transportation to/from appointments, and referrals to community services are often handled by case managers, even though these services may be out of the normal range of activities done by the case manager.

Determining Eligibility for Medicaid

When state/federal funding is requested to assist in paying for long-term care facility, receiving home, or community-based waiver services, the **financial records** of the individual will be examined by the state. Both real assets and income are taken into account, and any transfers for less than their fair market value will be questioned. The state "looks back" 36 months before the date the individual enters the facility or the date Medicaid is applied for. The look back can extend 60 months. Any transfer of assets for less than fair market value is subject to a **penalty period**, a period of time that a state will withhold payment for a nursing facility or other long-term care services. The penalty period is calculated by dividing the true worth of the asset by the average cost of the facility in that state. The following are the **exceptions to imposing a penalty period:**

- When the transfer was done to benefit a spouse.
- To certain disabled individuals or a trust for the individual.
- When the transfer was for a reason other than Medicaid qualification.
- When undue hardship would result from the penalty.

Trusts

A trust is property held by a person or trust company (the **trustee**) for the benefit of another (the **beneficiary**). The **grantor** is the person or entity that establishes the trust and puts in the assets. **Revocable trusts** allow the terms or beneficiaries to be changed and **irrevocable trusts** do not allow any changes in the terms or beneficiaries. Trust payments or amounts that could be paid to the individual in a medical/nursing facility are also treated as available resources in calculating Medicaid eligibility. Assets that cannot be paid or benefit the individual, but were transferred to the trust at less than market value to meet Medicaid eligibility, are subject to a penalty period during look back. The following **trust situations cannot be counted as available resources**:

- Set up by a parent, grandparent, guardian, or court for a disabled individual under 65 using the individual's own funds.
- Set up by a disabled individual, parent, grandparent, guardian, or court for a disabled individual, using the person's own revenues or pooled funds, managed by a nonprofit organization, and used for the sole benefit of each person included in the trust.
- Containing pension, Social Security, and other income of the individual, in states where individuals are eligible for institutional care under a special income level, but the trust does not cover the care for the medically needy.
- When the state determines that counting the trust would cause undue hardship.

Medicaid's Post-Eligibility Treatment of Income

Once an individual in a long-term care facility or nursing home is determined to be eligible for Medicaid, the **post-eligibility process** is used to determine how much the patient must contribute toward the cost of his or her care. To determine this amount, start with the monthly income of the patient and deduct the following:

- A personal needs allowance, which varies from state to state, but is at least $30.
- The community spouse's monthly income allowance, if the patient is married and the community spouse has insufficient income.
- An additional family monthly income allowance, if other family members reside with the community spouse.
- An amount for the medical expenses of the patient.

The amount remaining after these deductions is the amount that the individual is expected to contribute toward his or her cost of care.

Spousal Impoverishment Provisions

When a married patient is admitted to a long-term care facility or nursing home, the patient's spouse (the **community spouse**) usually remains living outside of the institution among the community. Under Medicaid's **spousal impoverishment provisions**, a portion of the couple's income is protected for use by the community spouse (i.e., it is excluded when determining how much the patient must contribute to their cost of care). The minimum amount of monthly income that is protected for the community spouse is $2,555 (July 2024 - June 2025, all states except AK [$3,192.50] and HI [$2,937.50]). The couple's income is divided into two categories: income earned by the patient and income earned by the community spouse. If the couple's combined income is more than the protected minimum, but the community spouse's income is less than the protected minimum, the patient's income is reserved for the community spouse to bring that spouse's income up to the protected minimum. There is also a maximum protected amount of $3,948 (2025). If the community spouse's income falls between the minimum and the maximum, that income is fully protected for the community spouse. However, if it is more than the maximum, the community spouse may be required to contribute a portion of the excess income to the care of the patient.

Public Sector Case Management

Public sector case management includes those patients on Medicare and Medicaid. Intervention and case management is targeted for high-risk pregnancy, high-risk newborns, sickle cell anemia, AIDS, psychiatric issues, cancer, and drug and alcohol patients. Working with this population presents challenges since there is often a lack of access to financial and transportation resources in order for the clients to help themselves. However, public sector individuals may have easier access to out-of-plan solutions since the system is flexible and review and approval by a payer is not required. A challenge for case managers is finding providers who will accept Medicaid payment, which is significantly lower than what private providers pay for services. The population also presents a challenge because elderly patients have multiple medical challenges, may be confused by the delivery system and associated processes, and may not take medications as prescribed due to financial restraints. An additional challenge is that support services to prevent complications from Alzheimer's disease are not covered.

Summary of Public Benefit Programs

	SSDI	SSI	Medicare	Medicaid
Benefits Offered	Supplemental income	Supplemental Income	Health insurance	Health insurance
Basis of Inclusion Criteria	Disability	Earnings; blind or disabled	Age; disability	Earnings
Funding	Federal tax revenues	Federal tax revenues	Tax revenues and premium payments	Federal and state tax revenues
Limits for Eligibility	N/A	Asset and income limits	N/A	Asset and income limits
Work Credits Required	Based on the age of disability	N/A	Medicare Part A requires 40 credits for free premiums	N/A

Military Benefit Programs

Military Healthcare Delivery System

The military healthcare delivery system is quite organized and highly well integrated. This system is comprehensive and usually thoroughly provides preventative healthcare services. The healthcare delivery system of the military is provided free to active duty military personnel in the United States Army, Navy, Air Force, Marines, and Coast Guard. Other uniformed nonmilitary personnel that may receive free health care in the military healthcare delivery system include certain members of the Public Health Services and the National Oceanographic and Atmospheric Association. **TRICARE** and the **VA system** provide the bulk of the military healthcare delivery system.

TRICARE

TRICARE is the health insurance program of the United States Department of Defense Military Health System. TRICARE was formerly known as CHAMPUS and functions by providing healthcare benefits and coverage to active duty personnel, National Guard and Reserve members, military retirees, their families, survivors, and certain former spouses of military personnel. It affords civilian health benefits to military personnel and their dependents. The plan offers comprehensive medical coverage, dental coverage, and special coverage by uniting the healthcare resources of the military with civilian networks of healthcare providers, hospitals and other facilities, pharmacies, and medical suppliers.

TRICARE for Life

TRICARE for Life is essentially a supplementary insurance for those who have Medicare A and B coverage and are eligible for TRICARE in the United States. TRICARE for Life serves as the primary insurance in overseas areas. Eligibility includes uniformed service members and families, National Guard, Reserve members and families, Medal of Honor recipients and families, survivors, former spouses, and others registered in the Defense Enrollment Eligibility Reporting System (DEERS).

VA Healthcare Program

The Veteran's Administration (VA) healthcare program is an integrated health care system that provides a number of different types of services for qualifying veterans, including those who were in the service during qualifying active duty dates and those currently in the service:

- **Medical centers**: Typical inpatient hospital treatment and surgery.
- **Preventive care services**: Periodic physical exams, immunization, genetic counseling, and health education.
- **Mental health services**: Inpatient and outpatient.
- Geriatrics, extended care, medical foster homes, domiciliary care, and state veterans' home: Provides long-term care in a variety of settings.
- **Hospice care**: Provides palliative care and grief counseling for patients and family members when the patient's life expectancy is 6 months or less and the patient is no longer receiving curative treatment.
- **Respite care**: Provides care to allow respite for caregivers.
- **Home health care**: Includes short-term skilled nursing services and homemaker/home health aide services.
- **Home telehealth**: Provides care coordination and remote monitoring of patients' conditions.
- **Homeless services**: Provided through medical centers and community-based partnerships.

CHAMPVA

CHAMPVA stands for the Civilian Health and Medical Program of the Department of Veterans Affairs. This is a comprehensive health program wherein the Veterans Administration shares covered supplies and healthcare costs with those eligible. CHAMPVA is run by the Health Administration Center located in Denver, Colorado, whereas TRICARE is a regionally managed program for active duty personnel, retired military personnel, military families, and survivors. To be eligible for CHAMPVA, a person cannot be eligible for TRICARE. Of note, CHAMPVA is the last payer after Medicare and other health insurance except for Medicaid, State Victims of Crime Compensation Programs, and supplemental CHAMPVA policies.

CHAMPVA for Life

CHAMPVA for Life provides VA healthcare benefits to family of veterans who were permanently disabled or killed in the line of service and who are not eligible for TRICARE. CHAMPVA for Life extends benefits to those 65 and older and functions as a supplementary insurance to Medicare. CHAMPVA for Life will pay for extended care service (with requirements similar to Medicare) but not for custodial care or assisted living. CHAMPVA covers hospice care and home health care for those who are homebound but does not cover adult day care. CHAMPVA covers inpatient mental health care for patients with advanced Alzheimer's disease but not long-term care.

Utilization Management Principles

Utilization Management

Utilization management has been in existence for more than twenty years. Early utilization management aspects involved focusing upon decreasing the number of inpatient admissions and decreasing or eliminating unneeded days in the hospital. Utilization management often involves healthcare plan administrators that review the medical necessity of hospital admission prior to the said admission (**precertification**) and who also decide if the ongoing and current care is appropriate (**concurrent review**). Utilization management is a prospective tool used to determine whether healthcare services are appropriate, medically necessary, and efficient. This is based upon established criteria, guidelines, evidence-based treatment plans, and provisions of the applicable health insurance benefit plan.

Characteristics of Utilization Management

Almost all utilization management systems use a **preadmission** or **precertification review** and **concurrent review**. Characteristics of the precertification review and concurrent review include data collection concerning diagnosis, appropriateness of rendered services, diagnostic test results, and symptoms. Review of criteria to validate services and conditions and evaluation of medical necessity are also characteristics of utilization management. Utilization management involves comparison of a patient's medical information to the established criteria of medical necessity. Case referral to a physician for review may be indicated in utilization management if it is determined that the criteria for medical necessity have not been met.

Utilization Reviews

Utilization reviews evaluate the need for services, the appropriateness of the services and the efficiency of those services. The reviews should support the need for the continuance or discontinuance of actions or interventions.

- **Preadmission** review allows documentation for the need for case management (3-5% of cases), rather than just acting as a census tool. It catches the unique aspect of each case and begins building the red flags needing resolution so that the case proceeds smoothly (e.g., notification to payer).
- **Concurrent** review shows the success or failure of treatments and provides the data for reducing lengths of stay or exploring alternative care plans. Concurrent review also documents the required processes for discharge success.
- **Retrospective** review allows the case manager to support their role in the treatment plan and provides valuable information in planning future, similar cases.

Coding Methodologies

Diagnostic-Related Group Codes

Diagnosis-related group (DRG) codes are essential for case management because the code assigned to the patient determines the reimbursement for care. The case manager has a number of responsibilities related to DRGs:

- Verifying that the correct DRG code has been assigned and that the code takes into consideration **complicating** or **comorbid** conditions (CC), **major complication** or **comorbid** conditions (MCC), or the lack of either.
- Remaining alert for and knowledgeable about CC/MCCs associated with different DRGs that may place the patient in a higher (or lower) DRG.
- Negotiating for a change in the DRG and length of stay (LOS) based on changes in diagnosis or treatment.
- Informing physicians and staff of working DRGs, anticipated length of stay and discharge date.
- Assisting in developing a plan of care that includes a target timeline, expected interventions, and patient outcomes.
- Monitoring for duplication of services or medical orders.

Current Procedural Terminology Codes

The case manager must be familiar with Current Procedural Terminology (CPT) codes, which cover outpatient procedures and durable medical equipment. Additionally, a number of CPT codes can be used to bill for conferences and consultations. These codes cannot be used for Medicare/Medicaid as they are status N (non-payable), but may be recognized by some insurance companies:

- **98966-98968**: Codes for telephone assessments and medical discussions ranging from 5 to 30 minutes if the patient has not been seen in the previous week or will not be seen within 24 hours (or next available appointment) of call.
- **99366** and **99368**: Codes for team conferences to discuss patient's care with or without the patient or family members present.
- **98969**: Code used for online medical assessment and case management services.

The Case Management Society of America is involved in lobbying efforts with CMS so that these codes are approved for CMS use. Beginning in 2015, CMS began paying for non-face-to-face coordination of care (code **99490**) for patients on Medicare with multiple chronic conditions.

Diagnostic and Statistical Manual of Mental Disorders Code

The Diagnostic and Statistical Manual of Mental Disorders, fifth edition, text revision (DSM-5-TR) is used as a guide for diagnosis of psychiatric and mental health disorders. It contains specific criteria that must be met for each diagnosis. The DSM-5 does not provide DSM diagnostic codes but includes the appropriate **ICD-10-CM codes**, although in some cases the ICD-10-CM codes are less specific than the DSM diagnoses, so different diagnoses may share the same code. For this reason, it's important that the health records document the **DSM diagnoses** and not just the ICD-10-CM coded diagnoses. The case manager should verify that diagnoses are correct (based on DSM criteria) and that the correct ICD-10-CM codes are used, as these determine the DRGs and rate of reimbursement. The case manager should also verify that ICD-10-CM Z codes, which can account for problems (such as family discord) that may affect patient outcomes and treatment plans, are properly applied.

Reimbursement Methods

INTERNATIONAL CLASSIFICATION OF DISEASES CODES

The International Classification of Diseases codes, ICD-10-CM for diagnoses and ICD-10-PCS for in-patient procedures, are used to determine the DRGs to which patients are assigned, and these determine reimbursement. The case manager must be familiar with ICD-10 coding in order to be a resource for other staff members to ensure compliance with documentation requirements, to carry out gap analysis, and to conduct impact studies.

- **ICD-10-CM***:* Codes comprise 3 to 7 characters of which the first character is alpha (all letters except U), second numeric, and fourth through seventh may be alpha or numeric. A decimal is placed after the first 3 characters. The first 3 characters indicate the diagnostic category, the next three characters indicate the etiology, anatomic site, or severity. A 7th character is an extension used to indicate external causes. Injuries are grouped by body part (for example, C15.3).
- **ICD-10-PCS***:* codes comprise 7 characters that provide information about 7 different items in order: section, body system, operation, body part, approach, device, and qualifier (for example, 0JHT3VZ).

For each patient encounter, the CPT code, ICD-10 code and diagnosis should be included. The case manager can access this information to guide their process. A sample **encounter form** is as follows:

Patient name:		File #:		Date:		Insurance:
√	CPT code	Item	Fee	√	Diagnosis	ICD-10-CM code
	99201	Minimal exam			Abd. Pain, unspec.	R10.9
	99202	Focused exam			Abscess	L02
	99203	Comp exam			Allergic reaction	T78.40

Negotiation Techniques

NEGOTIATION

Conflict in desires or needs between two or more people requires negotiation to reach a mutually satisfactory resolution. Case managers will often negotiate on behalf of their clients with insurance companies or providers of services. The goals of both parties need to be met. A successful negotiation occurs within a reasonable timeframe and without excess expense. The ability of both parties to comply with the agreement, as well as the predictable changes over time, are necessary for a successful negotiation to be workable and enduring. A successful negotiation does not necessarily mean all parties are happy with the outcome, however, it does mean an agreement is made within minimum time and expense that meets the true interests of the parties and establishes a basis of clear communication that fosters an environment for future, successful negotiations. A workable agreement allows both parties to meet their obligations within the time allotted. An enduring agreement has the ability to function successfully over the term of the agreement with enough flexibility to accommodate the variability of the patient's health, finances, and family situation.

SUCCESSFUL NEGOTIATION

Information is one key to successful negotiation; know the important factors for each circumstance. Keep focused on the patient. Remember **BATNA**: "best alternative to a negotiated agreement." This allows the case manager to explore alternate solutions rather than persisting in a negotiation that will not provide a desirable result. Both parties must trust the negotiator. **Trust** is built via good, timely communication and rapid action at times of agreement. **Respect** involves taking into consideration all parties involved in the negotiation, setting times and deliverables in a manner to takes into account everyone's schedules and circumstances. Avoid "irritators" during discussions. **Irritators** are terms that are judgmental or cause pain or embarrassment to either party. During negotiations, state specifics and facts without emotion or personal qualifiers. **Active listening** skills are essential to successful negotiations. Active listening includes understanding what is said and thinking about the content and implications of what is said. Active listening includes direct and indirect communications (e.g., body language, facial expressions, tone, and nuances of speech). **Repetition** of major points not only shows you have been actively listening, but clarifies the content and meaning of the discussion and allows exploration of possible alternatives.

UNSUCCESSFUL NEGOTIATION

The outcome of an unsuccessful negotiated settlement might have a win/lose result. "Getting the best of the other party" or "taking them to the cleaners" does not facilitate honest communication in future dealings. Persons or groups that feel they have been taken advantage of during negotiations may exhibit a lack of cooperation, anger, and inflexibility in future negotiations, even if the point of contention is minor and easily solved. Preconceived negative attitudes between the parties and with the case manager are established. Unsuccessful negotiations will not present future opportunities. Dealing with a vendor for one client may pave the way for others to benefit if the negotiation is successful.

Chapter Quiz

Ready to see how well you retained what you just read? Scan the QR code to go directly to the chapter quiz interface for this study guide. If you're using a computer, simply visit the bonus page at **mometrix.com/bonus948/ccm** and click the Chapter Quizzes link.

Psychosocial Concepts and Support Systems

Transform passive reading into active learning! After immersing yourself in this chapter, put your comprehension to the test by taking a quiz. The insights you gained will stay with you longer this way. Scan the QR code to go directly to the chapter quiz interface for this study guide. If you're using a computer, simply visit the bonus page at **mometrix.com/bonus948/ccm** and click the Chapter Quizzes link.

Abuse and Neglect

Types of Abuse

Seven types of abuse are listed below:

- **Physical abuse** is the physical use of force, and it can cause injury to the body, pain, or a form of impairment.
- **Sexual abuse** is any form of nonconsensual sexual contact.
- **Emotional abuse** is causing distress via verbal or nonverbal means. Isolation and lack of social interaction can be forms of emotional abuse.
- **Financial abuse** involves illegal utilization of money, assets, or property.
- **Neglect** is the failure or inability to provide obligations to the patient.
- **Abandonment** is the desertion of the caregiver who may have custody or who has taken on the care responsibilities of the patient.
- **Self-neglect** is an individual's behaviors that adversely affect the patient's health or safety.

Physical Signs of Abuse

Physical signs of abuse include bruises, contusions, cuts, black eyes, ligature marks, bone or skull fractures, open sores, punctures, burns, joint dislocations, unexplained sprains, broken hearing aids/glasses, medical evidence of underdose/overdose of medications, diarrhea or dehydration, fecal impaction, malnutrition, incontinence with evidence of rash, unkempt appearance/smell, lice, fleas, undergarments that are dirty/stained/bloody, absence of needed adaptive aids (prostheses, hearing aids, glasses), trouble with sitting/standing/walking, multiple ER visits or hospital admissions, sexually transmitted diseases/infections not explained by medical history, genital/anal trauma, patient's report of being mistreated physically/sexually/emotionally.

BEHAVIORAL SIGNS OF ABUSE OR NEGLECT

Being agitated/upset, fear of speaking, sudden behavioral changes, anger/irritation, depression, confusion/disorientation, unbelievable tales, marked changes in appetite/body weight, becoming quiet withdrawn/resigned, isolation, being uncommunicative, and patient's report of any emotional/verbal abuse are all **behavioral signs of abuse or neglect**.

OTHER INDICATORS OF ABUSE

- Discrepancy between income, assets, and lifestyle.
- Lack of explanation for inability to buy food and personal things and pay bills.
- The lack of assistance by caregivers/family members if the patient requires money for care, etc.
- Patient abandonment in a hospital, public areas or nursing home
- History of past abuse, mental illness, and drug or alcohol abuse in the caregiver or the patient.
- Caregiver not allowing patient to speak for herself or to be talked to without the caregiver being present.
- Obvious caregiver indifference, anger, or neglect directed at the patient
- Harassment, threats, or insults directed at the patient by the caregiver.
- Inability of patient to be seen without the caretaker present.
- Missed doctor's appointments and treatment delays.
- Varying accounts of injuries and incidents by the patient and family/caregiver.

Behavioral Change Theory

Change Agents

Any illness that affects an individual's life in physical, social, or psychological ways is considered a **change agent illness**. Change agent illnesses result in loss, anger, fear, anxiety, depression, dependency, and loss of self-respect, social status, or independence. **Catastrophic illnesses**, such as closed head or spinal cord injuries are easily recognized as change agents. Case managers must recognize that many cases fall into the category of "change agents" due to physical or psychological effects (e.g., a carpenter loses use of a hand or the main breadwinner can no longer function in that capacity). During the intake interview, it is important to document education, support mechanisms, counseling and/or medication that may be needed. Case follow-up needs to reassess the individual's success at coping with the illness and treatment as well as the effects on their family and community support group. Addressing the effect on the latter group maintains the patient's support group—the individuals providing social, psychological, and even financial support to the patient.

Stages of Change

Stages of change include the following:

Stage	Behavior
Precontemplation	The person is not yet ready to change their behavior and may not be aware of the need to change.
Contemplation	The person is getting ready to change their behavior (within six months); at this stage, the pros and cons are relatively equal.
Preparation	The person is ready to change and plans to implement changes within 30 days.
Action	The person has changed their behavior within the last six months but needs to focus on forward movement.
Maintenance	The person has achieved positive results and will need to strive to maintain these results.
Termination	The person has not returned to unhealthy behaviors/habits and has no desire or temptation to do so.

Transtheoretical Model of Change

The transtheoretical model/theory is also known as the stages of change model and determines a person's willingness to develop and act upon new and more healthy behavior. It also provides stages of change and strategies to enable a person to transition to action, maintenance, and resolution. James Prochaska and colleagues developed the transtheoretical model in 1977. This model involves four core concepts:

- Stages of change
- Change processes
- Decisional balance
- Self-efficacy

The health action process approach is a theory of health behavior change and involves a goal-setting stage and a goal-pursuit stage.

Behavioral Health Concepts and Systems

Behavioral Health Disorders

Approximately 25% of Americans suffer from some form of behavioral and mental health disorders. Up to 50% of patients with complex medical conditions, especially those with multiple diagnoses, will also have mental health or psychiatric problems that will have an influence on their recuperation and healing process. Case managers are instrumental in identifying the mental or behavioral issues that limit a patient's ability to attend to his or her healing, including attendance at rehabilitative sessions or follow-up appointments. Case managers have a responsibility to build their knowledge in psychiatric and behavioral health issues and treatments through attendance at workshops or seminars, reading books and journals, and building relationships with behavioral health professionals including social workers and psychiatrists.

Categories of Substance Use

Substance use can be described in three categories:

- **Substance use** includes using alcohol or drugs. Drug use may be legal or illegal and include synthetic or naturally occurring compounds.
- **Substance abuse** is the use of a substance either in an excessive or prohibited quantity that can cause deleterious effects to self, family, and others in society.
- **Substance addiction** is a physical and psychological compulsive need for an addictive substance and is considered a chronic condition with frequent relapses. It is characterized by three aspects: loss of control, compulsion, and negativity/anger when unable to obtain or use the substance.

Substance abuse and substance addiction are considered medical diseases and not character flaws. Frequently abused substances include alcohol, tobacco, cocaine, marijuana, amphetamines, hallucinogens, opioids, steroids, inhalants, and methamphetamine.

Dual Diagnosis

The term dual diagnosis is used with a patient who is both mentally ill and has substance abuse issues. This term may also be used to describe a person who suffers from an intellectual disability as well as a mental illness. The term may be used in a broad sense or in a restrictive sense. Determining a dual diagnosis may be quite difficult in substance abuse patients, as the substance abuse may in and of itself be a symptom of mental illness. It is important to differentiate between **pre-existing mental illness** and **substance-abuse-induced mental illness**.

Sexuality and Gender Identity

Sexuality is an integral part of each individual's personality and refers to all aspects of being a sexual human. It is more than just the act of physical intercourse. A person's sexuality is often apparent in what they do, in their appearance, and in how they interact with others. There are four main aspects of sexuality:

- **Genetic identity** or one's chromosomal gender
- **Gender identification** or how one perceives oneself with regard to male or female
- **Gender role** or the attributes of one's cultural role
- **Sexual orientation** or the gender to which one is attracted

Assessing and attempting to conceptualize a person's sexuality will lead to a broader understanding of the patient's beliefs and allow for a more holistic approach to providing care.

Gender Identity

Gender identity is the gender to which the individual identifies, which may or may not be the gender of birth (natal gender). Most children begin to express identification and behaviors associated with gender between ages 2 and 4. The degree to which this identification is influenced by genetics and environment is an ongoing debate because, for example, female children are often socialized toward classically female roles (dresses, dolls, pink items). Societal pressure to conform to gender stereotypes is strong, so gender dysphoria, which is less common in early childhood than later, may be suppressed. At the onset of puberty, sexual attraction may further complicate gender identity although those with gender dysphoria most often have sexual attraction to those of the same natal gender, so a natal boy who identifies as a girl is more likely to be sexually attracted to boys than to girls. Later in adolescence, individuals generally experiment with sexual behavior and solidify their gender identity.

Client Empowerment and Self-Care Management

Patient Advocacy

Acting as patient advocate is a primary role of the case manager. The need for a case manager comes from physical and emotional effects of the disease process or as a result of being overwhelmed by the quantity and complexity of the treatment plan. The case manager assists the patient and his family to attain self-determination and autonomy by empowering them with education about their disease, clarifying available options and services, explaining insurance benefits, community resources, and listening. The case manager has a legal and ethical responsibility to protect patients from misinformation and errors in comprehension. The case manager can obtain more information or clarification from providers. The case manager can also help the patient clarify their needs or wishes to their family and caregivers. The case manager has a major role in ensuring the patient's wishes are documented and observed.

Patient Activation and Patient Empowerment

Patient activation is the ability of the patient to express health concerns, to adequately question, and to develop skills needed to collaborate with healthcare providers. Patients should be encouraged to discuss concerns and should be guided in formulating questions: "What questions do you have?" and "What information do you need?" Patients should be assessed to determine their level of activation:

Level of Activation	Behavior
Level 1	Patient is overwhelmed and disengaged, remains passive and leaves healthcare providers in charge.
Level 2	Patient has increased awareness and can set simple goals but lacks adequate knowledge.
Level 3	Patient feels like part of the health team and begins to take action while building skills.
Level 4	Patient realizes the importance of self-management and remains goal oriented but may falter at times.

Patient empowerment is the ability of the patient to speak on his or her own behalf, to participate in healthcare decisions, and to manage personal healthcare to the maximal degree. Patient empowerment is often secondary to patient activation.

SELF-CARE MANAGEMENT

Self-care management involves active participation of the patient in his treatment of chronic illness or disability. The patient undertakes various activities to manage the daily impact of the condition. Such activities may include intentional actions or intentional inaction (i.e., doing nothing), taking control or taking responsibility for self, adopting coping strategies, managing emotions, setting goals, and changing behaviors. **Self-directed care** usually involves patient education, and such care needs to be based on the patient's perception of his illness/disability. A patient may have the tasks of evaluating his behaviors and daily activities and working on adopting health-promoting behaviors or activities. Other aspects include training in social skills and support, working with or without healthcare providers, and treatment compliance.

IMPORTANT FACTORS

There are many important factors in self-care management.

- Sometimes medical care and self-directed care can be seen as antagonistic strategies as opposed to synergistic strategies. It is important to utilize community resources and to understand the healthcare organization to maximize healthcare delivery support as well as decision support.
- The patient should be viewed as a key resource in goal setting and problem solving in the development of new skill sets.
- The patient should also have dynamic input in the development of new health-oriented behaviors.
- It helps to enhance self-care and medical care if patients with a chronic illness or disability can work with families and healthcare providers.

INFORMED DECISION-MAKING AND SHARED DECISION-MAKING

Different models of decision-making include the **paternalistic/maternalistic model** in which the healthcare provider assumes to know best and makes decisions, but this can result in unwanted treatment. Another model is the **sovereignty model** in which the client makes the decision about the care that the client wants, regardless of whether the client lacks the necessary knowledge to make an informed decision. These models have evolved into the **shared decision-making model** in which the client and healthcare providers work together to reach a decision that is in the best interest of the client. The healthcare providers provide a thorough explanation of all proposed treatments and interventions as well as the associated risks and benefits. The client should be made aware of all options and provided information about possible complications, increased morbidity, or risk of death. The client should participate by asking questions and reviewing the information in order to reach an appropriate decision.

OUTCOMES OF SELF-DIRECTED CARE

The outcomes a patient has when establishing self-directed care may include health restoration and disease prevention. Lifestyle changes and optimal level of health maintenance may be the result of illness or disability limitation. Such changes could include those undertaken by patients, their families, and their children to stay active and meet personal mental and physical health goals. This may involve treating an acute condition and could also involve meeting psychological and social needs. A patient should also be cognizant of trying to prevent minor accidents or illnesses and any long-term issues. A patient with such issues should attempt to maintain his health and well-being after an exacerbation or admission to the hospital by needed lifestyle changes and maintenance of a pleasing quality of life.

Outcomes of Self-Advocacy and Self-Management

Self-advocacy and self-directed care have been shown to decrease pain, enable shared decision making about treatment, and to enable a sense of control in a patient's life. It has also demonstrated a decrease in the frequency of visits to healthcare providers and an increase in perceived quality of life. Such self-care involves the activities of daily living and modifications that enable the patient to keep chronic issues under control and to decrease the effect that such issues have on his physical health status and his daily functioning. It also enables the patient to deal with the psychological aspects of the chronic illness/disability. For example, a patient that suffers from heart failure and who opts for self-care may choose to adjust his diet, adhere to a medication regimen, and exercise every day. He can also seek help when symptoms happen or treat exacerbations before they get severe by monitoring his weight daily.

Examples and Barriers

There are many ways to be involved in self-advocacy and self-directed care such as aerobic exercise, cognitive symptom management and self-reliance to manage personal symptoms/illness. Such skills can decrease the number of ER visits and hospital admissions for the chronic illness or disability. Internet-based educational modules that allow a patient to access his own medical records and enter data can help to improve self-care skills. Self-advocacy and self-directed care emphasize the magnitude of the ability to access support for decisions for patients. Some barriers to this skill set may include personal barriers, inability to relate to healthcare providers, and lack of access due to cultural biases and social deprivation.

Community Resources

Definition, Goals, and Examples of Community Resources

Community resources are a collection of assistance programs or services provided to community members. Such resources may be organizations serving a certain geographical area or certain groups of people. Typically, the goal of community resources is to positively impact **community growth** and to improve the **quality of life** of community members. These resources may be at no cost or at low cost and may be run by the government, local businesses, or other community members. Some examples include fraternal/religious organizations, government programs, pharmacy assistance programs, educational organizations, and financial assistance organizations.

Early Childhood Intervention Programs

Early childhood intervention programs target infants and children (0 to 6 years) who have been victims of or are at risk for abuse and/or neglect or have developmental delays. Federal, state, and local programs are available with some authorized by the **Individuals with Disabilities Education Act (IDEA)** specifically for infants and children who are diagnosed with mental or physical conditions that may result in developmental delay. **Healthy Families America** is a home visiting program designed to educate and support expectant and new parents in order to prevent abuse and neglect and promote the well-being of the child and family. Early childhood intervention programs attempt to provide the resources necessary to promote optimal development. Early intervention programs may supply equipment and services, screening (such as for hearing/vision deficit), parent education, mental health counseling, diagnostic services, nursing services, nutritional services, therapy (occupational physical, psychological), and social work services. Some children need a wide range of services, and these are coordinated by a case manager who ensures the child receives the needed services.

Religious and Fraternal Organizations

A **religious organization** is a nonprofit entity that does one of the following: conducts worship, supports religious activities of nonprofit organizations, or propagates the tenets/teaching of religious faiths. Religious organizations are typically organized around a shared religious belief and may include various benefits. Benefits may include mutual aid and assistance to those in need. Examples would include the Aid Association of Lutherans, American Friends Service Committee, Faith and Light, and Missionaries of Mary.

A **fraternal organization** is an organization implying a formal fraternity or brotherhood. Examples include the Knights of Columbus, Loyal Order of Moose, Sons of Norway, and Sons of the American Revolution.

Government Programs

Government programs were initially established in the United States during the 1930s as a result of the Great Depression. Such government programs usually involved welfare payments, Medicaid health care, Food Stamps, provisional aid to pregnant women/young mothers, and federal and state housing benefits. Government programs are considered to be a means of social protection. Such programs are usually created to enable those in need to overcome adverse conditions. Government programs vary widely from state to state and from nation to nation. Some examples of government programs include substance abuse and mental health services, SSI/disability services, emergency food assistance, and Medicaid.

Resources for Transportation

A case manager can arrange transportation for patients who are so infirm that assistance is required to/from healthcare facilities (from one hospital to another) due to medical necessity. Coverage by health plans is not usually available from a healthcare facility to the patient's home. Wheelchair vans or ambulette services may be used for stable patients or those with their own oxygen who do not need it regulated by a professional. Wheelchair van transportation is rarely a covered benefit. **Ground transportation ambulances** are generally two types: 1) basic life support (BLS), which includes limited monitoring by a BLS paramedic and 2) advanced life support (ALS), which includes an ALS paramedic, cardiac monitoring, and a drug box. This is the most common transportation between acute care and rehabilitation hospitals. **Air ambulances** provide advanced cardiac life support (ACLS) personnel, cardiac monitoring, and a medication box along with a registered nurse. Unless arranged by a case manager, air transportation is usually not covered by health plans; exceptions may be transportation from an inaccessible region (e.g., mountaintop) or speeding to a hospital for an approved organ transplant.

Pharmacy Assistance Programs

Pharmacy assistance programs often are conducted by pharmaceutical companies to enable patients to obtain their medication free or at low cost. These companies may provide **discount cards** and/or **waivers** to aid uninsured or low-income patients with purchasing medication. Some pharmacy assistance programs are conducted by or through the state. Currently, twenty-eight states have pharmacy assistance programs for seniors and other groups. Twenty-two states solely fund state pharmacy assistance programs, and six states utilize waiver programs that are funded by both the federal and state governments via Medicaid.

Conflict Resolution and Crisis Intervention

Reasons for Conflict

There are multiple reasons for conflict. Some reasons include an unresolved crisis, unrealized need for power or attention, the perception of an inability to succeed, and an unrealized need for physical or emotional safety. Another cause of conflict may involve **boundary issues**. Boundary issues may include a lack of boundaries, undefined or unclear boundaries, boundaries that are not enforced, boundaries that allow excuses, or boundaries that are violated. One method to decrease or prevent conflict is to continually assess the existing power structure and how the power structure facilitates the needs of the members for safety, success, and power.

Boundary Setting in Conflict Resolution

One useful strategy in conflict resolution is that of setting boundaries. Boundaries facilitate a win-win power structure and foster cooperation and respect while creating an environment that is success oriented. Setting boundaries also enables outcomes, either positive or negative, to happen in a nonpunitive setting. Boundaries function more effectively than rigid rules in that rigid rules usually originate from a power source and often foster a win-lose environment. It is important to clearly state the boundary and its limits before it is violated. Other elements involved in setting boundaries include listening, negotiation, and empowerment.

Effective Communication in Conflict Resolution

Effective communication is a vital element in conflict resolution. Direct communication with the person involved in conflict reduces complications by the avoidance of complaining and of triangulation. Ensure that the communication is not from a reactive or an emotional stance. Reactivity often fuels conflict. Another effective communication strategy is to focus on the presenting issues. When focusing on the presenting issues, it is important to leave emotions and feelings out of the discussion. If emotions or feelings are impeding resolving the conflict, it is important to deal with them away from the situation in a neutral environment.

Other Strategies in Conflict Resolution

Some of the other strategies in conflict resolution include the formation of a win-win **power dynamic** or **authority relationship**. This dynamic can be achieved requesting and listening to the input of other team members. By requesting input from the other team members, they will feel validated and empowered and will help to create a positive work environment and facilitate goals. It is also important in resolving conflict to ensure that the environment is success oriented by establishing concise and clear goals. If the team environment has become reactive and thus a source of conflict, the environment should be restructured to one that is proactive.

Crisis Intervention Strategies

The goals of crisis intervention strategies include producing **improved** levels of functioning for the patient, returning the patient to a **pre-crisis** level of functioning, and preventing the patient from settling for **suboptimal** levels of functioning. Approach the patient with an optimistic attitude and offer hope. Offer encouragement, but do not promise or guarantee an outcome. Attempt to stay event-focused, and allow the patient to express feelings and frustrations. Analyze and attempt to mobilize the patient's support system. Try to enable the patient to begin coping again by helping him focus on an immediate task.

Family Assistance During Crisis

Families of patients must deal with the effect of the patient on the normal operation of their family life. Realignment of family responsibilities occurs each time someone suffers from illness or injury, and prolonged illness puts unique burdens on family dynamics. It is important for the case manager to understand the family dynamics and provide **intervention resources** when needed. If the family was fractured before the illness, chances are the fracture will intensify, causing problems in addressing the treatment plan of the patient. To assist families through periods of crisis, a case manager can suggest family counseling or support groups for the family or the caregiver; recommend books on the illness or coping with the illness; direct families to sources for financial assistance; remind the family that maintenance of their regular routines, appointments and activities is important to their physical and psychological health; and encourage the family to communicate with one another.

Adaptive and Maladaptive Families

An **adaptive family** is able to adapt to a crisis, specifically a catastrophic illness, with flexibility, reasonable problem solving, effective communication between the family and the care providers, and the ability to maintain their link to the community. When a family cannot continue with their own daily functions while meeting the patient's needs, they are a **maladaptive family**. Maladaptive actions include overindulgence of the patient and/or abandoning other family members, denial of the patient's condition, relying on a single person to provide all assistance to the patient, and failure to seek assistance or accept help from others. Case managers must assess the family/support group at the start and throughout the course of an illness by asking probing questions to make sure they understand the scope of the situation. The connection between the family and community resources may determine the level of involvement necessary by the case manager to ensure the best result is achieved for the patient.

Health Coach

A health coach basically serves as a personal medical trainer. Coaches may work with patients who have chronic illnesses and help to provide information about lifestyle changes and services that are available. A health coach can be a nutritionist, nurse, or a health educator. Coaches are trained to help patients identify health risks and to motivate them to change their behaviors to bring about a healthier lifestyle. A health coach may also provide information regarding medical conditions, concerns, or issues. Some may even suggest questions that a patient might ask at the next doctor visit. Health coaches form a team with the patients and help them to set manageable goals and provide positive reinforcement.

Interpersonal Communication

INTERPERSONAL COMMUNICATION

Interpersonal communication is the process by which individuals articulate ideas, thoughts, and feelings to other individuals. **Direct interpersonal communication** implies a face-to-face interaction between the individual that is sending the message and the individual that is receiving the message. Direct interpersonal communication involves messages between individuals who are in an interdependent relationship. Due to the fact that direct interpersonal communication involves immediacy (i.e., it occurs right now) and primacy (i.e., it occurs right here), it typically will create strong feedback. Interpersonal communication includes **verbal** communication as well as **nonverbal** communication. Interpersonal communication may be categorized by two different means.

CATEGORIES OF INTERPERSONAL COMMUNICATION

The concept of interpersonal communication may be described by the number of participants, by the function of the communication, or by the location of the communication.

- When interpersonal communication involves two people, it is considered **dyadic communication.**
- **Group interpersonal communication** involves three or more people and typically serves to problem solve or to make decisions.
- **Public interpersonal communication** involves a large group and typically functions to share information, to provide entertainment, or to persuade.
- **Organizational interpersonal communication** is interpersonal communication that occurs in a large organization; an example might be communication between an employer and a worker.
- **Family communication** would be an example of utilizing setting to categorize interpersonal communication.

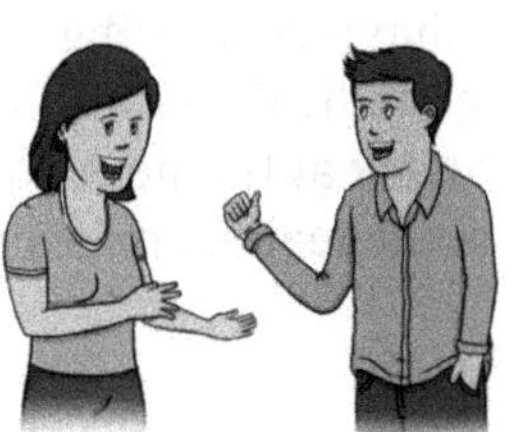
Dyadic Communication

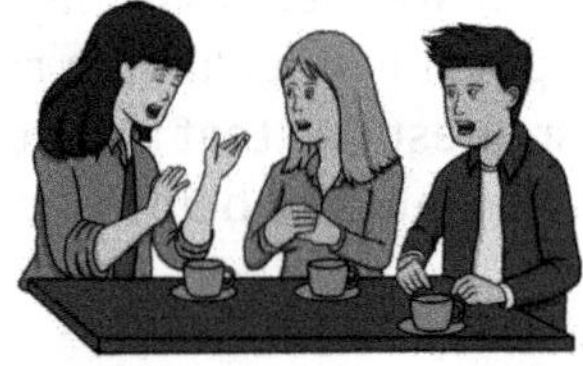
Group Interpersonal Communication

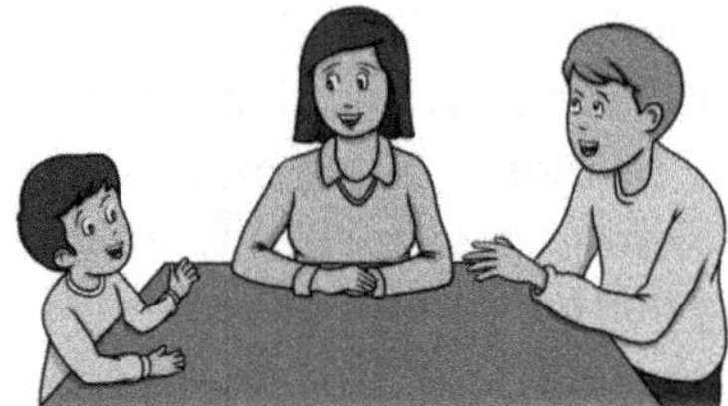
Family Communication

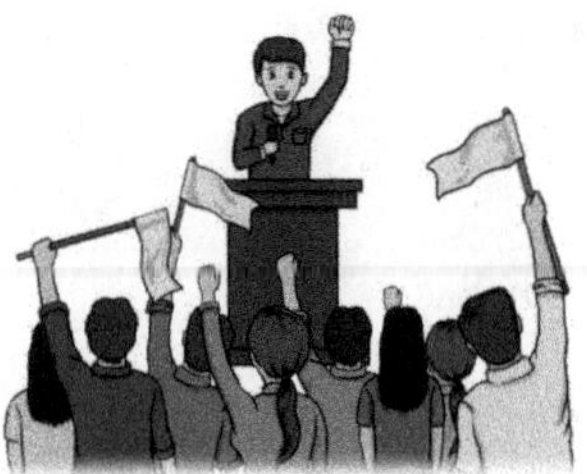
Public Interpersonal Communication

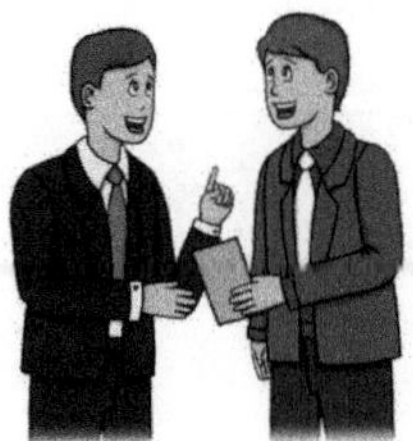
Organizational Interpersonal Communication

Barriers to Good Communication

Barriers to good communication include the following:

- **Physical interference** occurs when the client is distracted by the physical surroundings. Optimal communication occurs in a quiet space without distractions.
- **Psychological noise** occurs when the client is thinking about something else. This could be pain, hunger, anger, or the issue of payment for services. Be sure the client is as comfortable as possible and explain that services are part of their benefit package and are at no additional cost.
- **Information overload** is caused by an abundance of information or by cognitive, intellectual, or educational deficits. Notice the client's eye contact, ask questions to assess the client's understanding, and use vocabulary the client understands.
- **Perceptual barriers** block your message or filter the information. These occur based on the client's unique experiences, cultural background, education level, or value system.
- **Structural barriers** are caused by layers of bureaucracy or communication the client or their family deals with. Written communication between the clinical team and client insures clarity for all involved.

Role and Function of Interpreters

Interpreters have a vital and often overlooked role and function in healthcare management and delivery. Interpreters enable the patient to communicate effectively with healthcare providers and also enable the patient to have a clear understanding of the medical system. Interpreters also serve to assist the healthcare team in providing the patient with information about the medical condition and treatment options. There are no licensing requirements for interpreters or accreditation requirements. Some interpreters may obtain training in medical terminology to facilitate interpretation in the healthcare setting. Many interpreters are informal native speakers and often function on a volunteer basis.

Health care agencies that are federally funded are required to provide **free interpretive services** for clients speaking commonly encountered foreign languages. The patient must be informed that an interpreter will be made available to them. In order to ensure appropriate care and communication, a third-party interpreter who is trained in medical terminology, fluent in both languages being used, and familiar with the ethics and HIPAA regulations of acting as an interpreter is the best option. Meeting these requirements ensures compliance with federal guidelines. Family members cannot be required to serve as interpreters unless the client specifically requests a family member to act in this capacity.

Communication Between Case Manager and Physician

Focused and conscious communication between case managers and physicians must be established and maintained. It is important for case managers to use medical terminology in their communications with physicians and for the physician to realize the case manager can provide education and support services to their patients. Often the case manager role is not understood by physicians since they are brought into the case after initial treatment has started. Physicians often lack insight into the social and environmental aspects of the patient; case managers provide this insight. Power struggles occasionally occur in care planning since decisions by physicians are often made from a different agenda than case managers' decisions; the case manager's role must be made clear to the physician. Physicians may not be aware of limited policy coverage or lack of community support once discharge takes place. Case managers provide this information and assist in the discharge or care plan creation.

Group Dynamics

Group dynamics is the study of the interactions between members of a group and is also utilized as a broad term to denote group processes. A group is typically defined as two or more people that are connected by social relationships. Groups adopt many dynamic processes that distinguish them from a random collection of individuals due to interaction and influence. The dynamic elements involved include norms, roles, relationships, development, the need to belong, social influences, and behavioral effects. In organizational group dynamics, the concept of the group process is relative to the behavior of the members of a group whose task is to problem-solve or to make decisions.

Interviewing Techniques

It is important to utilize many techniques when conducting an **assessment interview**. Interview techniques may include questions to use, questions to avoid, styles of communication to avoid, specific age variations to consider, emotional variations to consider, and cultural variations to consider.

- The **open-ended question interview technique** is useful to obtain information on the client's feelings and the client's perceptions. Example: Tell me about your relationship with your spouse?
- The **close-ended question technique** is useful to gather facts and to obtain specific information from a client. Example: How long have you been married?
- The interview technique of using a **laundry list approach** (in which a question is asked and then a list of words/options to answer the question is provided for the patient to select from) elicits specific answers. This technique also facilitates an in-depth pursuit of data that deviate from normal. Example: What word best describes your relationship with your spouse? Loving, open, comfortable, secure, necessary, frustrating, unhealthy, volatile, or empty.

Communication Styles

Interview techniques rely on excellent communication skills and communication styles. Communication styles to avoid include poor eye contact or using too much eye contact, multitasking during the interview or being too physically removed from the client, asking questions that are biased or leading in nature, rushing the client, and reading the interview questions from a form. Interview techniques also need to consider specific age variations. For example, when conducting an interview with a pediatric patient, all the information will need to be validated by a responsible family member.

Variations in Interview Techniques

The interview technique should take into account **emotional and cultural variations**. Emotional variations would include angry, anxious, depressed, or manipulative clients. Angry clients would require the following interview techniques: a calm, reassuring, and controlled approach; allow the client to express his feelings; provide the client with personal space; and avoid argument. With an anxious client, the interview technique would be a simple and organized informational approach that explained the purpose of the interview. The interview technique to use with a manipulative client would be one that provided structure and set boundaries and limits.

Health Literacy Assessment

A health literacy assessment is the determination of a patient's ability to read, comprehend, and utilize information related to health care to make informed decisions and to follow treatment plans. More than 50% of patients cannot comprehend even basic healthcare information. A low score on a health literacy assessment reduces treatment success and furthers the chance of medical error. At the very least, health literacy involves the basic need to understand and to be understood. Health literacy skills include communication with healthcare providers, reading and comprehending health information, medication information and compliance, instructions on the use of medical devices, and understanding information on various treatment options.

Multicultural, Spiritual, and Religious Factors

Cultural Competence

Culturally competent behavior goes beyond knowing general facts; it is a dynamic process of being aware and showing respect for cultural differences of all types. It begins with being aware of one's own beliefs and not letting them interfere with the care provided. Just as each case manager brings his or her own individual background, beliefs, and practices to the caring experience, each patient and family have their own unique contributions to the care plan. **Cultural competence** is providing competent care that corresponds with the patient and family's own cultural background. The case manager provides a complete and unbiased, sensitive assessment of the patient's background and beliefs, obtains further knowledge as necessary, then coordinates and executes a plan of care that is meaningful to the patient and family, regardless of the care provider's own beliefs.

Patient's Belief System

Currently, almost 14% of people living the US are foreign-born, over 22% speak a language other than English at home, and others speak little or no English at all. This presents case managers with clients having diverse cultures, religions and other factors that present barriers or issues in developing treatment plans. Case managers must understand the patient's attitudes toward accepting treatment from healthcare providers since their knowledge of illness, health, and healing may be based in custom rather than science. **Cultural idiosyncrasies** must be taken into account in creating treatment plans that will be followed and thus successful. For instance, some cultures believe home death is desirable. Through education, case managers can become aware of the cultural needs of the community they serve.

Respect for Cultural Diversity

The case manager should first assess his or her own background, values, and beliefs in order to consciously avoid biases. It is helpful to obtain further knowledge in order to understand the background being addressed and to show acceptance of differences even when they may diverge from his or her own comfort zone and culture. A case manager should also acknowledge differences concerning end-of-life care, be sensitive, and be open to the individual patient's beliefs rather than trying to predict behavior. Assumptions regarding care, needs, or beliefs should **not** be made based on race or ethnicity.

CLAS Standards

The CLAS standards are primarily directed at health care organizations; however, individual providers are also encouraged to use the standards to make their practices more culturally and linguistically accessible. The principles and activities of culturally and linguistically appropriate services should be integrated throughout an organization and undertaken in partnership with the communities being served. The 15 standards are organized by themes: Culturally Competent Care, Language Access Services, and Organizational Supports for Cultural Competence. Within this framework, there are three types of standards of varying stringency: mandates, guidelines, and recommendations as follows: CLAS mandates are current federal requirements for all recipients of federal funds. CLAS guidelines are activities recommended by the Office of Minority Health (OMH) for adoption as mandates by federal, state, and national accrediting agencies. Culturally and Linguistically Appropriate Services (CLAS) in Health Care are offered by the US Department of Health and Human Services (HHS) Office of Minority Health National Standards.

Impact of Spirituality on Health Behavior

Spirituality has been linked to health behaviors. Studies show that patients who are spiritual have fewer **self-destructive behaviors** such as suicide, smoking, and alcohol or drug use. All major religions promote the idea that the body is a gift from God or a higher power/spirit and prohibit self-destructive behaviors. Spirituality has been demonstrated to lower blood pressure, decrease depression, and to boost the immune system. Some religions, however, may prohibit certain forms of medical care, such as Jehovah's Witnesses refusing blood transfusions. Spirituality also enables a patient to have additional social support and improved coping skills through prayer. Studies show that spirituality affects mental health by providing a patient with optimism, increased coping ability, and a sense of a greater purpose.

Neuropsychological Assessment

Elements of Neuropsychological Assessment

Neuropsychological assessment was historically used to determine the extent of functional skill loss a person had sustained due to injury or illness affecting the brain, as well as the specific location(s) in the brain that had been affected. As a field, it has evolved into the measurement of brain dysfunction relating to language, attention, concentration, memory, and perceptual and motor skills. The primary components of a neuropsychological assessment are taking the patient history, interviewing the patient, and administering one or more standardized assessments. Two examples of commonly used neuropsychological assessment instruments are the Luria-Nebraska Neuropsychological Battery, used to measure organic brain damage and the location of injury and the Bender® Visual-Motor Gestalt Test, which measures brain dysfunction.

Assessment Tools for Patients with Impairments

The case manager's **assessment** must include temporary or permanent functional changes; physiological, psychological, or social problems; possible problems functioning in the community; and educational deficits of the patient and family. Although observation is the initial tool used, a variety of test results may be needed to arrive at a diagnostic conclusion including independent medical evaluation, personal interviews, and detailed review of all psychiatric records. The Minn. Multiphasic Personality Inventory, Ranchos Los Amigos Levels of Cognitive Functions, and Glasgow Coma Scale are assessment tools used frequently in initial and continued assessment of a patient. The results of the tests assist the case manager in designing the **individualized plan for placement** of the patient and the level of services needed. Stroke, brain trauma, and spinal cord injuries/lesions patients require vastly different treatment plans and equipment depending on the location and extent of the problem. Family members may not have formal testing, but their level of cognition must be noted in the case file in order to create an individualized plan for the patient.

Ranchos Los Amigos LCF Assessment

The following are the **Ranchos Los Amigos Levels of Cognitive Functioning** scoring criteria:

I	**No Response**	Totally unresponsive to all stimuli.
II	**Generalized Response**	Inconsistent or non-purposeful reactions; delayed reaction to deep pain stimuli.
III	**Localized Response**	Specific but inconsistent reactions; reaction in a manner not related to the stimuli.
IV	**Confused/Agitated**	Short attention span, confusion, excited behavior, impaired speech, tires easily, no cooperation in the treatment plan.
V	**Confused/Inappropriate**	Alert and responsive to simple commands and familiar people, needs structure, may wander, and may have memory impairment.
VI	**Confused/Appropriate**	Goal-directed behavior but needs structure, aware of environment, has the ability to learn but needs frequent repetition.
VII	**Automatic/Appropriate**	Follows a daily routine but cannot deal with unexpected situations, vague understanding of their condition but no real cognition of the details or the future.
VIII	**Purposeful/Appropriate**	Alert and oriented, functioning within confines of the current injury, understands a skill once learned without supervision, able to function in society unless an unexpected or stressful situation occurs.

Psychological Elements of Illness and Disability

Chronic illness is an illness or disorder that lasts for an extended period or may be permanent and affects a patient's ability to lead a normal life. **Disability** is defined by the ADA as "a physical or mental impairment that substantially limits one or more of the major life activities of the individual, a record of such an impairment, or a situation in which an individual is regarded as having such an impairment." Many factors contribute to the **psychosocial aspects** of chronic illness and disability. Such factors include the degree of functional limitations, the decreased ability to undertake the activities of daily living, the decreased capacity to perform one's life roles, indefinite prognosis, and the extended need for medical treatment and possible rehabilitation. Other aspects include stress, both psychological and social, of the illness or disability itself; the resulting impact on relationships with family and friends; and possible prolonged financial stressors such as decreased income or increased medical bills. Some basic concepts of the psychosocial aspects of chronic illness and disability include stress and the disturbance of social, psychological, and behavioral balance. Loss, grief, distortion of body image, stigma (stereotypes/prejudices), possible uncertainty of the course of the illness/disability, and changes in quality of life are all aspects to be considered.

Social Determinants of Health

Social determinants of health include:

- **Socioeconomic status**: Income needed to pay for medications, doctor visits, and treatments
- **Transportation availability**: Private vehicle or public transportation
- **Food security**: Sufficient income to purchase adequate food and availability of grocery stores and food markets in close proximity to home
- **Housing**: Homeless status, adequate or inadequate housing
- **Support systems**: Family, friends, and neighbors who know the client and can provide support in some way
- **Education**: Level and quality of education and job training
- **Employment**: Employed full or part-time or unemployed, salaried or piecework
- **Neighborhood**: Safe or high crime area; availability of stores, churches/mosques/temples, markets, and healthcare facilities; exposure to trash-filled streets; presence or lack of parks and recreational areas; residential segregation or integration
- **Exposure to violence and crime**: Exposure to gangs, criminal elements, drug dealing, domestic/intimate partner violence
- **Social attitudes**: Racism, sexism, bigotry, ageism, tolerance, acceptance
- **Language and literacy**: Ability to read, write, and comprehend, fluency in English
- **Health literacy**: Level of knowledge regarding anatomy, physiology, and healthcare

Supportive Care Programs

Support Groups

A support group consists of members that are united because of an illness, disability, cause, or issue. The group is usually **nonprofessional** and may function to provide information, share personal experiences, provide empathy, suggest resources, and lend a listening ear. Some examples include addiction, Alcoholics Anonymous, AIDS, Alzheimer's, anxiety disorders, and many others. Some support groups meet in person, while others may be online. Some support groups are operated by professionals who do not have the illness, disability, or issue shared by the members. Such professionals may serve as moderators for discussion or offer other managerial services.

Support groups include pastoral counseling, disease-based organizations, and bereavement counseling. **Support groups** may have various aspects to render support and assistance. Some aspects of support groups/programs may include financial, emotional, and practical support and may also extend to family members, caregivers, and healthcare providers involved in the patient's care.

Disease-Based Support Groups

The American Diabetes Association, American Cancer Society, American Heart Association, National MS Society, and National Kidney Fund are examples of **disease-based organizations**. Such organizations provide support in the form of educational resources and may also provide suggestions for community resources or financial resources for patients. Some other little-known disease-based organizations include the Accu-Chek Patient Assistance Program (provides Accu-Chek test strips to patients with diabetes), American Cancer Society Hope Lodges (provide lodging for patients or their families), American Kidney Fund Health Insurance Premium Program (financial help for insurance premiums for patients requiring dialysis), and numerous other disease-based programs also exist.

Bereavement Counseling

Bereavement counseling is a type of **psychotherapy** that helps a person deal with grief or mourning after a loss. Such a loss may be the death of a loved one or a major life event that causes loss, such as a traumatic accident, diagnosis of a life-threatening illness, diagnosis of a chronic illness, or disability. Bereavement counseling is indicated when a patient becomes extremely stymied and overwhelmed with his grief and loss and loses his ability to use normal coping skills. Counselors also help the patient with other issues such as insomnia, vivid dreams, poor concentration, and appetite loss. A bereavement counselor strives to guide the patient to think of positive solutions or thought processes concerning his loss and may suggest **coping strategies**.

Pastoral Counseling

Pastoral counselors are trained professionals and have training in both psychology and theology. They provide **spiritual and psychological support** and guidance to patients and families in the healthcare environment. Pastoral counselors may conduct religious services, perform religious rites, and lend companionship as well as counseling to patients and families. They also may work with medical professionals to instruct them about ethical and spiritual issues and to explain various religious beliefs and practices. Another role for the pastoral counselor is to aid medical professionals in assuring that the patient has his emotional and spiritual needs met. A degree in pastoral counseling usually requires a bachelor's degree, a three-year professional degree from a seminary, and/or a master's or doctoral degree in a mental health field.

Wellness and Illness Prevention

The Wellness Concept

The wellness concept is a balanced model in which the body, spirit, and mind must **coexist** in harmony. Such a concept indirectly came from the Eastern philosophies of Buddhism and Taoism that suggest that mind, body, and spirit join together as one. Wellness was defined in the 1950s by Dr. Halbert Dunn. Dr. Dunn defined wellness as "an integrated method of functioning which is oriented toward maximizing the potential of which the individual is capable of functioning within the environment." The wellness concept has six elements of health: **physical**, **emotional**, **intellectual**, **social**, **spiritual**, and **vocational**. The extent to which a patient internalizes the concept of wellness and takes personal responsibility determines his success in obtaining wellness.

Wellness Strategies

Wellness strategies are often called the health triangle. The **health triangle** incorporates physical, emotional, and social wellness concepts.

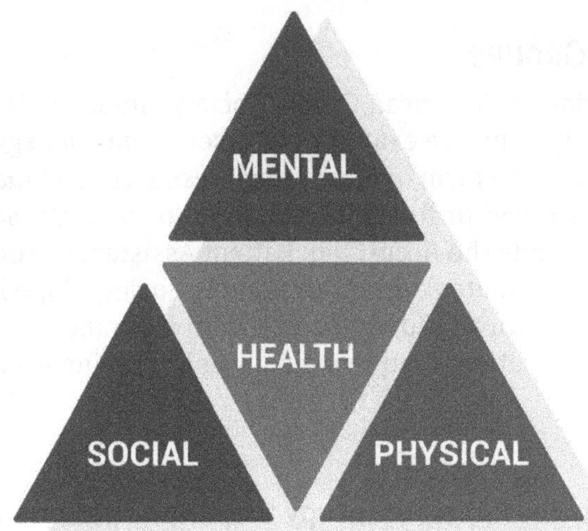

- **Physical wellness strategies** include exercise and fitness, nutrition and diet, lifestyle choices/habits, safety, medical self-care, and health screening. Currently, many companies and employers are implementing wellness programs in the workplace. Such programs may include nutrition seminars, tobacco cessation, and the importance of physical activity and exercise in maintaining health and wellness.
- **Emotional wellness strategies** include stress control, expressing feelings, problem solving, assessment of personal limitations, outlook-optimism/pessimism, recognition of successes/failures, maintaining a sense of humor, and understanding and recognizing the consequences of one's actions.
- **Social wellness strategies** include interaction with other people and the environment, instigating and maintaining relationships, and participation in various groups/social causes.

Additional Wellness Strategies

More and more, it is being realized that wellness not only involves physical, emotional, and social aspects but also involves integrating strategies for intellectual, spiritual, and vocational wellness to achieve an optimum wellness balance.

- **Intellectual**: Lifetime learning, using the mind, investigating new ideas, making decisions, following directions, and maintaining speaking and listening capabilities.
- **Spiritual**: Developing purpose and meaning in life, connecting with one's higher power, prayer, meditation, morals/ethics, and contemplating one's death.
- **Vocational**: Goal setting, learning new skills, identifying abilities, determining personal goals/missions, and volunteering.

Illness Prevention

The illness prevention concept focuses upon disease prevention by reducing the risk of a disease, identifying possible risk factors, or by detecting disease at an early stage in order to facilitate treatment. Strategies include immunizations; well-baby/child checkups; calcium and vitamin D supplementation to decrease the risk of osteoporosis; screening exams for breast, colorectal, and prostate cancer; and monitoring blood pressure and cholesterol.

Chapter Quiz

Ready to see how well you retained what you just read? Scan the QR code to go directly to the chapter quiz interface for this study guide. If you're using a computer, simply visit the bonus page at **mometrix.com/bonus948/ccm** and click the Chapter Quizzes link.

Quality and Outcomes Evaluation and Measurements

Transform passive reading into active learning! After immersing yourself in this chapter, put your comprehension to the test by taking a quiz. The insights you gained will stay with you longer this way. Scan the QR code to go directly to the chapter quiz interface for this study guide. If you're using a computer, simply visit the bonus page at **mometrix.com/bonus948/ccm** and click the Chapter Quizzes link.

Data Interpretation and Reporting

Data Interpretation in Case Management

Data interpretation in case management entails establishing connections and comparisons and exploring causality and subsequent results. The **relevance** of the findings includes the following: does the indicator satisfy the target? is the indicator far from the target? how does the indicator compare to established data? and do extreme variations exist in the data? Possible reasons for the findings need to addressed by research into expert opinions and by considering the use of routine service data. Examples of routine service data may include a calculation of the nurse-to-client ratio or a review of product data versus client load.

Cost-Benefit Analysis

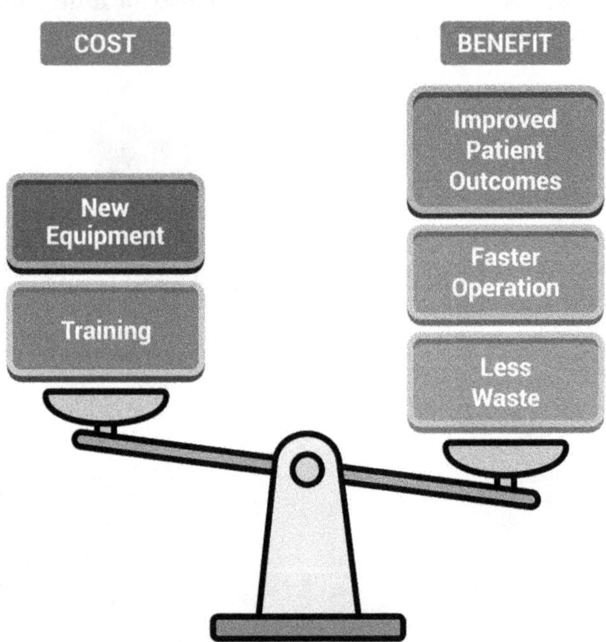

Attaching value to the job of a case manager is an important aspect of their role. Case management adds cost to a program, but costs that are, hopefully, offset by savings. At a minimum, **cost-benefit reports** should contain an overview and summary of case management intervention; any fees attached to the case management tasks; actual charges and the savings, both gross and net; and the status of the case being reported. Potential savings should be documented and although they are difficult to quantify, these segments of the case need to be included in order to present a complete picture of the case. When a case manager works for a client (HMO or self-insured employer), it is recommended that a cost-benefit analysis of their case load is submitted every quarter. **Quarterly reporting** allows a manageable amount of information to be processed and the effectiveness of services to be reviewed on a timely basis that allows for adjustments to the plans, if necessary. Be aware that cost-benefit analysis reports are often used by the marketing and quality assurance departments of organizations.

CASE MANAGER REPORT

Initial and subsequent case manager reports need to sell the management plan and its role in problem solving, outline the cost savings due to case management, and address any anticipated objectives available due to creative, analytical thinking. The interest of the patient must predominate. The report must present an **objective view** while meeting the unique **requirements** of the entity receiving the document. Besides containing the main points of why the client came into the case manager's care, the report must contain information about the payer source(s), medical history and current physicians, a review of policy coverage and limitations, and community resources and alternative treatment programs. Make sure all recommendations are presented as to their ability to meet the patient's needs and present provider information about their quality of services and ability to meet patient needs. A presentation on the costs of treatment should be included in a separate section so it does not appear as an influence to recommended services.

END OF SERVICES SURVEY

At the conclusion of a case, especially an involved or long-term relationship case, it is important to provide the client with a **satisfaction survey**. The survey or questionnaire must be as objective as possible. The survey results assure clients that case management does make a difference to the families receiving the services. The results affirm that the services provided are those needed by the recipients of the services. Responses are a tool used to train professionals, meet the needs of patients, and respond to the expectations of payers. The public relations and marketing departments also appreciate the results of user surveys.

Health Care Analytics

HEALTH RISK ASSESSMENT

Health risk assessments are tools used to assess an individual's health risks. A number of different tools are available, but they usually include a questionnaire and metrics that provide a score that is used to determine the degree of risk. Some health risk assessments are targeted toward specific populations, such as older adults or those with diabetes. The results should be provided to the individual as part of developing a plan of care. Most health risk assessments include questions about the following:

Category	Data Collected
Demographics	Age, sex, address, income
Lifestyle	Diet, exercise, substance abuse, gambling, absenteeism, seatbelt use
Medical History	Personal, familial
Vital Signs	Pulse, respiratory rate, temperature, blood pressure, pain level, oxygen saturation, weight, height
Screenings	Mammogram, cholesterol, CBC
Psychological Status	Depression, anxiety, confusion, psychiatric screening

Both Medicare (annual physical) and Medicaid (enrollment physical) utilize health risk assessments. Health risk assessments are useful in determining risks as well as predicting the need for and the costs of interventions.

Predictive Modeling

Predictive modeling (predictive analytics) utilizes datamining and statistics to develop a model that predicts outcomes. Once a problem is defined, data (often derived from medical records and insurance claims) is gathered about the problem area or population and analyzed with software (machine learning) and different models are proposed to solve the problems. These models are then assessed and ranked according to their likelihood of success and the best model is then tested. For example, if predictive modeling suggests that a certain type of patient is at high risk for complications, then the model may provide alerts about potential risks when the patient's data is entered into the system so that healthcare providers can take steps to moderate the risks. Predictive modeling, which can include social factors as a part of analytics, can help to identify individuals who have an increased risk for readmission because of health and/or social challenges.

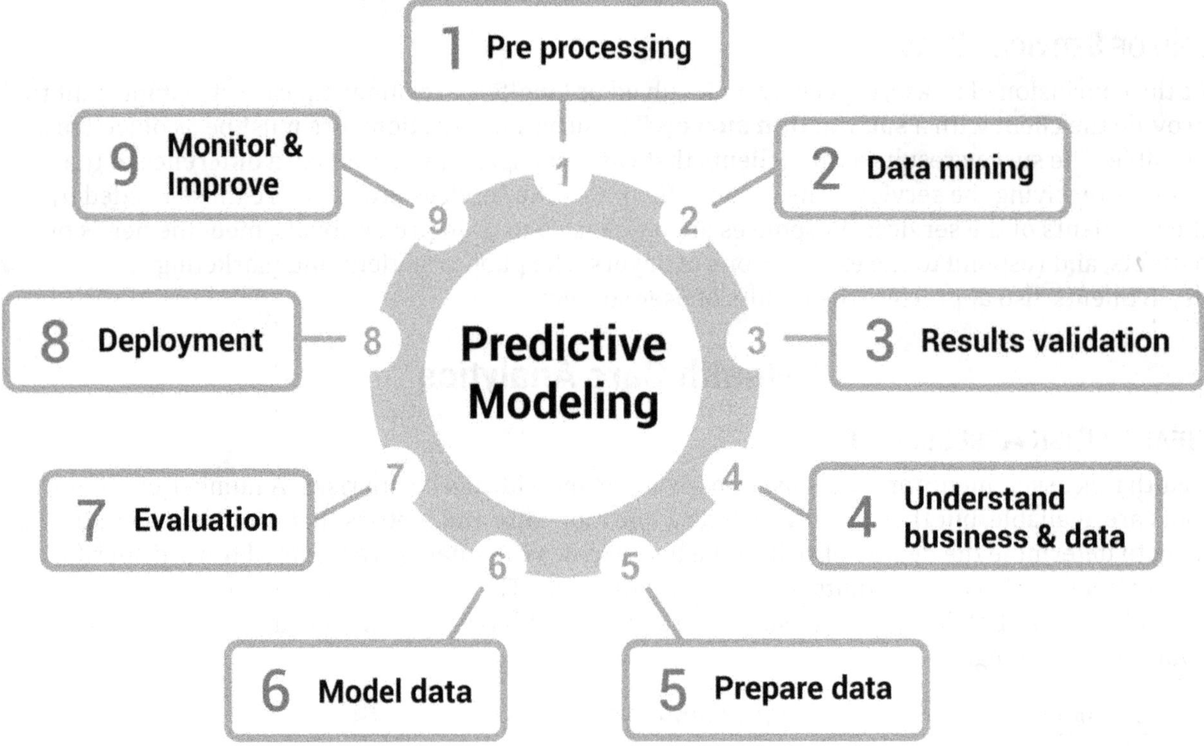

Caseload Calculation

In general, the caseload in case management has been inconsistent and inappropriate with regard to its size. Some organizations have attempted to design methods of **caseload calculation** to enable case managers to accurately determine appropriate caseload. Many of these methods have focus or application limitations. Also, the rapid evolution of the case management arena, such as adding utilization management and disease management into the tasks of case management, has created more difficulty in establishing reliable benchmarks for determining caseload. The Case Management Society of America (CMSA) and the National Association of Social Workers have published a **Caseload Concept Paper** as a result of their collaborative efforts to provide a means to determine caseload calculation.

Caseload Matrix

The caseload matrix is a schematic made up of four categories that comprise factors that affect the complexity and the size of a caseload.

- The first category is the **initial factors** that impact the caseload. Such factors are the business environment, segment of the market involved, legal and regulatory requirements, setting of the clinical practice, characteristics of individual case managers, medical management services, and technological support.
- The second category is the comprehensive needs assessment.
- The third category is the **case management interventions** that are required.
- The fourth category is the **outcomes**—short, intermediate, and long term.

Length of Stay

Length of stay (LOS) is determined by the number of days a patient is hospitalized for a single episode of care, beginning with the date of admission and excluding the date of discharge, so a patient admitted on October 4 and discharged on October 9 would have a LOS of 5 days. Long-stay patients are those with LOS of 7 days or more. The prospective payment system in which Medicare pays according to DRG has encouraged healthcare organizations to reduce LOS because longer than anticipated LOS's do not receive additional reimbursement. **Average length of stay (ALOS)** is based on the average of patients' length of stays. The ALOS may be calculated on a weekly, monthly, or annual basis for an organization as a whole or may be calculated according to unit or service area. The national ALOS is published by Medicare and is currently 4.5 days. AHRQ provides data regarding LOS through its **Healthcare Cost and Utilization Project (HCUP)**, based on data from payers, including Medicare, Medicaid, and private insurance companies.

InterQual

InterQual, a product of McKesson, provides support for clinical decisions through a number of different products that aim to improve patient outcomes and facilitate care management:

Level of care criteria	Guidance in selecting appropriate level of care criteria for acute care, acute pediatric, acute rehabilitation, long-term acute care, subacute and SNF, home care, outpatient rehabilitation and chiropractic.
Care planning criteria	Promotes quality and cost effective criteria for special treatment and molecular diagnostics and provides SIM*plus*, a risk-management tool.
Behavioral health criteria	Focuses on providing evidenced-based criteria for psychiatric conditions, substance abuse, and dual diagnosis with criteria available for seniors, adults, adolescents, and children.
Coordinated care content	Focuses on high-risk and complex cases to provide more efficient care, reduce costs, provide evidence-based care, and meet regulatory requirements.
Evidence-based development	Provides research into evidence-based practice.

The goals of InterQual include preventing over- and under-utilization, reducing risks, facilitating communication, improving data collection, supporting consistency of care in alignment with CMS guidelines, reducing costs, identifying areas in which improvement can be made, facilitating payments, and identifying trends.

Adjusted Clinical Group System

The Adjusted Clinical Group (ACG) System was developed by John Hopkins University. ACG provides tools for healthcare organizations to measure morbidity and identify patients who are at high risk and to predict utilization of healthcare services in order to set equitable rates for reimbursement for care. ACG includes case-mix classification that allows comparison of different patient populations. The patient's diagnostic codes are assigned to one of the 32 different **Aggregated Diagnosis Groups (ADGs)**, so that one patient may be assigned more than one ADG. Diagnoses are assigned to an ADG based on:

- Condition duration (acute, chronic, recurrent) and length of predicted care.
- Condition severity.
- Certainty of diagnosis and whether or not further diagnostic services will be needed.
- Disease etiology (injury, infection, other).
- Need for specialty care, such as surgery, obstetrics, or oncology.

The patient will then be assigned to one of the 102 **ACG categories** based on the patterns of the ADGs, considering clinical judgment and data analysis.

Program Evaluation

Program evaluation is essential in case management. Program evaluation involves analyzing the utility of the program and the direction of the program. Such evaluation is vital to program planning, budgeting, and program management. Program evaluation gives insight into what elements of the program are working well and what elements may not be working well. Accountability is also a function of program evaluation. This function allows a manager to determine if the program is truly meeting the needs of the designated patient population in the manner intended. Program evaluation also facilitates long-term planning for the healthcare system.

Outcome Measures

Outcome measures is defined as the outcome of a patient's health status as a result of health care provided. Outcome measures may be used to judge the impact that the provided healthcare services had upon achieving the desired outcome for the patient. These measures also may yield information on the cumulative effect of multiple elements of health care and also may yield information on certain care areas that need quality improvement. Examples of outcomes measures may include in-hospital mortality, readmission rates within thirty days, medication errors, infection rates, emergency department visits after hospital discharge, and health status of a patient two weeks' post discharge.

Quality and Performance Improvement

Key Terms

- **Palliative care program** is the process of continual assessment of a patient's needs and their treatment options in accordance with the patient's values and beliefs.
- **Continuous quality improvement** (CQI) is a key module of total quality management using a meticulous, systematic, organization-wide methodology to achieve ongoing improvement in the quality of healthcare services and operations. CQI looks at both outcomes and processes of care.
- **Efficacy of care** is the potential, capacity, or capability to achieve the preferred outcome or effect of treatment as previously defined by scientific or research-based findings.
- **Integrated delivery system (IDS)** refers to a single organization or a group of affiliated organizations providing a wide variety of ambulatory and tertiary care and services.

Quality Improvement

The concept of quality improvement is based upon the following principles for improvement: health care has to be safe, effective, patient-centered, efficient, equitable, and delivered in a timely fashion. **Continuous quality improvement** is a management philosophy that contends that most services can be improved. In health care, continuous quality improvement has a strong emphasis upon the healthcare organization and system. Quality improvement focuses on objective data to analyze and improve healthcare processes.

Core Concepts and Steps of Quality Improvement

The core concepts of quality improvement are the following:

- Quality involves meeting or exceeding client expectations.
- Achievement of success in quality improvement is manifested by meeting the needs of the client.
- Most of the issues result from the processes not the individuals involved.
- Reducing or eliminating variation in processes decreases variations in outcomes.
- The scientific method should be used to implement incremental changes.

The **core steps** in quality improvement include team formation with knowledge of the improvements needed in the system, definition of specific goals and needs of clients, identification and definition of improvement, and implementation of strategies for change to produce improvement.

Performance Improvement

The concept of performance improvement is a method of improvement that came from realizing that poor performance of a job is rarely due to a lack of knowledge or skills but is usually due to other factors in the system. Performance improvement is defined by the International Society for Performance Improvement as "a set of methods and procedures, and a strategy for solving problems, for realizing opportunities related to the people. It can be applied to individuals, processes, and organizations. It is, in reality, a systematic combination of three fundamental processes: performance analysis, cause analysis, and intervention selection."

Core Concepts of Performance Improvement

Some of the **core concepts** in performance improvement are the following:

- Consideration of the institutional environment.
- Identification of gaps between the actual performance and the desired performance.
- Determination of causality of gaps in performance.
- Implementation of solutions designed to decrease or eliminate the gaps in performance.
- Measurements of performance change.
- Identification of future training needs with the introduction of new job tasks, new equipment, or new techniques with the assumption that performance will decrease when jobs change.

Core interventions in performance improvement include mentoring, supervision, documentation, staff selection, and team building.

Quality Indicators

Types of Quality Indicators

Quality indicators are measures used to determine the quality of healthcare provided. The case manager is responsible for developing and implementing quality indicators, which include:

Indicators	Aims
Clinical	Those aimed at evaluating the effectiveness of clinical care and assessing the safety of patients. These may include assessing patients for risk of falls or risk of suicide as well as following policies and procedures related to discharge and follow up of clients.
Financial	Those aimed at assessing the cost-effectiveness of interventions. These may include reviewing rehospitalizations and comparing the outcomes of different interventions and their associated costs.
Productivity	Those that assess the amount of work accomplished, often used to evaluate the time needed to manage a case and then using that data to determine caseload.
Utilization	Those that assess which services are most used and least used, and how this relates to client outcomes. Utilization indicators are used as part of utilization review to assess whether treatment provided is medically necessary.

Agency for Healthcare Research and Quality

The Agency for Healthcare Research and Quality (AHRQ) is one of the agencies in the United States Department of Health and Human Services. The AHRQ functions to improve American health care in the areas of quality, efficiency, and effectiveness. Information gathered by research of the AHRQ is designed to aid individuals to make informed healthcare decisions and to improve the quality of American health care. AHRQ has the following areas of focus: comparison of treatment effectiveness, patient safety and quality improvement, health information technology, prevention and care management, and healthcare value.

AHRQ Clinical Quality Indicator Modules

Clinical quality indicators (QIs) are those indicators that are evidence-based and used to measure the quality and safety of health care. Clinical quality indicators were developed by the Agency for Healthcare Research and Quality (AHRQ) under their patient safety and quality improvement initiative. AHRQ provides free software for hospitals to use to collect data. **AHRQ quality indicator modules** include:

Quality Indicator	Focus
Prevention	Use discharge data to determine those who need preventive care after discharge.
Inpatient	Use discharge data to determine quality of care through quantifying mortality data, procedure volume, and treatment under or over use.
Patient Safety	Use discharge data to determine the potential for adverse events and complications.
Pediatric	Use discharge data to determine the quality of pediatric care, including rates of screening, preventive efforts, and iatrogenic complications.

Patient experience is the total of all experiences the patient has as a part of the provision of healthcare. This can include the patient's expectations, problems, and rate of satisfaction. Quality indicators are all aimed at improving the patient experience.

Patient-Centered Outcomes

The research of the AHRQ in the area of patient-centered outcomes provides data on the most effective medical treatments for a given condition based on current scientific information and comparisons of current treatments or methods to deliver health care. Such comparative research enables patients to understand the most effective treatment and the inherent risks of such treatment. AHRQ has an evidence-based practice center program, which offers contracts to facilities in the United States to produce types of evidence-based reports. These EPC reports are available to be viewed on the AHRQ website.

National Quality Strategy

The National Quality Strategy (led by AHRQ for the HHS) aims to improve the quality of healthcare and promote the sharing of best practices throughout health services on the local, state, and national level through the following:

- **Three aims** (to guide and assess efforts to improve healthcare): Better care (patient-centered), healthy people and communities (utilizing proven interventions), and affordable care.
- **Six priorities** (to help to achieve aims): Proving safer care (reducing harm), encouraging collaboration (engaging clients/families), ensuring effective communication/coordination of care, promoting effective prevention efforts and treatment (especially for leading causes of disease), using best practices to promote healthy living, and making care affordable (through new models of healthcare).
- **Nine levers** (to align with the NQS): Measurement and feedback; public reporting; learning/technical assistance; certification, accreditation, and regulation; consumer incentives/benefit designs; payment (incentives, rewards); health information technology; innovation/diffusion; and workforce development.

National Committee for Quality Assurance

The National Committee for Quality Assurance is an influential nonprofit accreditation organization whose goal is to improve the quality of healthcare through the use of evidence-based research. NCQA works closely with state and federal agencies in developing healthcare policies. NCQA promotes the **measure-analyze-improve-repeat formula** for quality improvement and has tracked steady improvement annually.

Services include accreditation for health plans, physicians, provider organizations, and other organizations, including case management accreditation. **Certification programs** include disease management, utilization management and credentialing, and multicultural health care. **Recognition programs** focus on programs that utilize current clinical protocols and deliver quality healthcare, including practice and clinical programs. NCQA has developed the **Patient-Centered Medical Homes Recognition program**, whose standards guide the change to this model of patient care management. NCQA ranks and reports on health insurance plans, and NCQA currently accredits health plans that provide coverage for over 90% of Americans. NCQA developed the **Healthcare Effectiveness Data and Information Set (HEDIS)** as performance measures that allow consumers to compare health plans. Most health plans collect and report HEDIS data, and Medicare requires HEDIS data for HMOs.

UTILIZATION REVIEW ACCREDITATION COMMISSION

URAC (Utilization Review Accreditation Commission) is a nonprofit organization that provides accreditation to healthcare organizations to facilitate quality health care. The goal of URAC is to encourage continued improvement in quality and efficient healthcare management via education and accreditation. URAC is a nonprofit entity and is therefore not controlled by specific investors who may have a stake in a URAC process. Also, the board of directors of URAC is comprised of those representing the following: consumers, healthcare providers, employers, regulators, and experts in industry.

ACCREDITED HEALTH CARE ORGANIZATIONS

URAC awards accreditation to numerous healthcare organizations. Such healthcare organizations include medical management entities, health insurance plans, hospitals, and health Web sites. **Medical management organizations** include disease management, case management, medical call centers, and independent review organizations. The accreditation and review process involved in obtaining URAC accreditation requires a policy and procedure review coupled with an on-site visit to the organization. The on-site visit assures that the applying organization is actually complying with its stated policies and procedures. Once the review is completed, URAC will determine the accreditation status.

ACCREDITED PROGRAMS

URAC has numerous accreditation programs. Some of the URAC accreditation programs are Case Management, Credentials Verification, Health Network, HIPAA Privacy, Pharmacy Benefit Management, Workers' Compensation Utilization Management, Claims Processing, HIPAA Security, Provider Performance Measurement and Public Reporting, Workers' Compensation Property and Casualty Pharmacy Benefit Management, Consumer Education and Support, Drug Therapy Management, Health Provider Credentialing, Specialty Pharmacy, Health Utilization Management, Mail Service Pharmacy, Uniform External Review, Comprehensive Wellness, Health Content Provider, Medicare Advantage Deeming Program, and Workers' Compensation Health Network. The **accreditation standards** are created for URAC by an expert committee that is comprised of people that represent different healthcare interests in the healthcare arena.

CASE MANAGEMENT ACCREDITATION

Case management is a rapidly expanding healthcare practice area. Healthcare organizations are realizing that case management aids in improvement in meeting a patient's healthcare needs and also aids in the improvement of treatment outcomes. Case management achieves such improvements by the coordination of the full healthcare spectrum. URAC provides accreditation to a multitude of organizations involved in case management to aid in ensuring that the case management is of high caliber and meets URAC standards. URAC **standards of case management accreditation** include the following: staff structure and organization, information management, quality improvement, and complaints.

NATIONAL QUALITY FORUM

The National Quality Forum (NQF) is a nonprofit organization that utilizes a threefold mission statement in its goal of improving American healthcare quality. The NQF operates by the mission of "building consensus on national priorities and goals for performance improvement and working in partnership to achieve them, endorsing national consensus standards for measuring and publicly reporting on performance, and promoting the attainment of national goals through education and outreach programs." NQF members include consumer organizations, physicians, nurses, hospitals, supporting industries, private and public purchasing agents, and quality improvement organizations.

Structure and Standing Committees

The National Quality Forum is governed by a **board of directors** that manages the entire organization and utilizes a specific focus on certain strategic policy issues. The board is made up of members that represent major stakeholders from both the public and private arenas. The National Quality Forum has multi-stakeholder, volunteer committees to expedite its processes and make the organization transparent. There are more than 20 ongoing standing committees with one of the most recent being the disparities standing committee.

The **Consensus Standards Approval Committee** functions to review all consensus standards that have been recommended or endorsed by the National Quality Forum. The members of this committee utilize expertise in healthcare quality improvement and performance measurement.

The **Health IT Advisory Committee** functions to give the NQF current guidance regarding its health information technology portfolio and provides expertise on certain health information technology projects. Such projects include **eMeasures** testing requirement specifications and quality data set maintenance.

Member Councils

The membership of the National Quality Forum is organized under eight member councils that function to advise the Board of Directors and to advise the standing committees. The eight member councils are:

- The Consumer Council
- The Health Plan Council
- The Health Professionals Council
- The Provider Organizations Council
- The Public/Community Health Agency Council
- The Purchasers Council
- The Quality Measurement, Research, and Improvement Council
- The Supplier and Industry Council.

Each of the eight member councils of the National Quality Forum functions to give different insights on improving healthcare quality and building an accepted consensus.

Joint Commission Standards and National Patient Safety Goals

The **Joint Commission Standards** are those that are used as the basis of evaluation for accreditation for healthcare organizations. For example, the standard on medical record security requires that healthcare organizations comply with HIPAA regulations and ensure privacy and security of records. The Joint Commission publishes standards on many different aspects of care and management. The case manager, as part of performance and outcomes management, may monitor and report compliance with Joint Commission standards.

The Joint Commission also develops and updates the **National Patient Safety Goals (NPSGs)**, whose overreaching goal is to improve patient safety. The case manager must be aware of the NPSGs that apply to different program types. Current NPSGs are tailored for ambulatory health care, behavioral health care, critical access hospitals, home care, hospitals, laboratories, long-term care, nursing care centers, and office-based surgery. As part of the NPSGs, the Joint Commission provides a list of look-alike/sound-alike drugs and a "Do not use" list of abbreviations.

CMS Core Measures

Core measures are the evidence-based use of treatments to reduce the risk of complications. CMS publishes **core sets** (groups of core measures) of clinical quality measures (CQMs) each year. 2025 core measure sets include:

Core Measure	Clinical Quality Measures
Primary Care Access and Preventative Care	Adults: Cervical cancer screening, chlamydia screening, flu vaccinations, screening for depression, breast cancer screening Children: Weight assessment and counseling for nutrition and physical activity, immunization status, well-child visits, developmental screening in first three years of life
Maternal and Perinatal Health	Adults: Elective deliveries, prenatal and postpartum care, contraceptive care Children: Audiological diagnosis no later than 3 months of age, live births weighing < 2,500 g, low-risk cesarean deliveries
Care of Acute and Chronic Conditions	Adults: Controlling high blood pressure, comprehensive diabetes care, diabetes short-term complications admission rate, COPD or asthma in older adults admission rate, heart failure admission rate, asthma in young adults admission rate, all-cause readmissions, asthma medication ratio, HIV viral load suppression Children: Emergency department visits for children, asthma medication ratio
Behavioral Health Care	Adults: Substance abuse/dependence treatment, medical assistance with smoking and tobacco use cessation, anti-depression medication management, follow-up after hospitalization for mental illness, diabetes screening in people with schizophrenia or bipolar on antipsychotic medications, use of opioids at high doses in persons without cancer, concurrent use of opioids and benzodiazepines, use of pharmacotherapy for opioid use disorder, follow-up after ED visit for mental illness, adherence to antipsychotic medications Children: Follow-up for children prescribed with ADHD medication, monitoring for children on antipsychotics
Dental and Oral Health Services	Children Only: Percentage of eligible individuals that receive preventive services, sealant receipt on permanent first molars
Experience of Care	Adults and Children: Consumer assessment of healthcare providers and systems (CAHPS) health plan survey
Long-Term Services and Supports	Adults Only: National core indicators survey (NCIDDS-AD); Percent of members >18 years of age with documentation of a long-term service and support (LTSS) care plan

CMS is currently working with other health plans to align and simplify core measures. The goal is to have quality measures that improve patient outcomes become aligned so that there is less complexity in reporting.

Clinical Quality Measures

Clinical quality measures (CQMs) are tools utilized to measure and monitor the quality of healthcare services provided by healthcare providers, hospitals, and critical access hospitals in such aspects of patient care as health outcomes, safety, cost-effectiveness, clinical processes, coordination of care, and patient engagement and adherence. Healthcare providers who participate in CMS electronic health record (EHR) incentive programs must submit CQM data through certified EHR technology. CMS establishes updates to CQM specifications each year.

Evidence-Based Care Guidelines

Critical Pathways

Critical pathways are also known as care paths, critical paths, and clinical pathways. Critical pathways are management and care coordination plans that create goals for a patient and give the progression of **mechanisms** to accomplish such goals with an optimum of efficiency. Critical pathways have become important in healthcare management as a means to standardize medical care, decrease inefficient use of resources, reduce healthcare costs, and to hopefully improve medical care quality. These pathways serve as a tool to provide the details of the medical care processes and to uncover inefficiencies within the processes.

Goals

Some of the goals of critical pathways include choosing the optimum practice when the existing practice varies in an unnecessary fashion, delineating standards for length of stay and for appropriate utilization of diagnostic tests and medical treatments, scrutinizing how various levels/steps in the medical care process interrelate and more efficiently coordinating such steps, providing common goals for hospital personnel to enable such personnel to understand and efficiently facilitate their collective roles in the entire process of a patient's medical care, provide data to educate healthcare providers on variations from an expected medical outcome, decrease redundant documentation, and improve patient satisfaction.

Clinical Guidelines and Protocols

Clinical **guidelines** differ from clinical pathways in that clinical guidelines are consensus statements that are created in a systematic manner to enable a healthcare provider to make management choices that are based upon the patient's unique medical circumstances. Clinical guidelines may be utilized in the creation of critical pathways but are not routinely addressed in critical pathways.

Clinical **protocols** are treatment regimens or treatment recommendations that are a result of clinical guidelines. Some clinical protocols may be somewhat similar to critical pathways in that their goal may be to standardize treatment.

Chapter Quiz

Ready to see how well you retained what you just read? Scan the QR code to go directly to the chapter quiz interface for this study guide. If you're using a computer, simply visit the bonus page at **mometrix.com/bonus948/ccm** and click the Chapter Quizzes link.

Rehabilitation Concepts and Strategies

Transform passive reading into active learning! After immersing yourself in this chapter, put your comprehension to the test by taking a quiz. The insights you gained will stay with you longer this way. Scan the QR code to go directly to the chapter quiz interface for this study guide. If you're using a computer, simply visit the bonus page at **mometrix.com/bonus948/ccm** and click the Chapter Quizzes link.

Adaptive Technologies

Assistive Devices

Assistive or adaptive devices are products that allow an individual to be more independent in performing activities when they have impaired abilities or functional limitations. The devices may be used on a temporary basis during treatment or they may be a long-term solution following reasonable effort to learn the task. The assessment for use of an assistive device is similar to the overview needed for use of durable medical equipment. Assistive devices include the following categories: visual aids (glasses, audio books); hearing aids; speaking/communicating devices (text-to-voice synthesizer); orientation to time/place/person (memory books, clocks); ambulation/location (cane, walker, wheelchair); eating (nonskid mat for plates, rocker knife); dressing (button hook); toileting (toilet seat with rails, bedside commode); shower/tub (grab bars, tub chair, hand-held nozzle); transfer (gait belt, hydraulic lifts for bed/chair/stairs); and recreation (large print books, video games, fishing pole harness). The patient and caregivers need to be involved in the selection of the device and understand its use. Documentation for the need of the device must be provided by the case manager for the insurance provider to cover the costs.

Assistive Technologies

Assistive technology involves both devices and services. An **assistive technology device** is any technology item utilized by patients with disabilities to perform tasks/functions that may otherwise be quite arduous or impossible and thus enables greater independence. An **assistive technology service** is any service that helps a disabled patient in the choice of a device, the acquiring of an assistive technology device, and in the use of an assistive technology device. Examples of assistive technology devices include canes, walkers, wheelchairs, scooters, specialty keyboards, trackball mouse, joystick, and the Teletypewriter. Assistive technology services examples are computer services, blind and low-vision services, ergonomic, and business modification services.

Various Adaptive Technologies

Adaptive technologies include:

- **Teletypewriter (Telecommunication device for the deaf) (TTY/TDD)**: Special typewriter-like device with a small screen that allows the hearing impaired to type and receive a message that is transmitted over telephone lines. Both the sender and receiver must have the device installed.
- **Electronic travel aids**: Devices that emit energy waves to help the visually impaired individual detect objects in the environment through audible or tactile signals. The device may be incorporated into canes, such as the Laser cane and Ultra cane.

- **Electronic orientation aids**: The individual aims a receiver at a transmitter of a talking sign, and the person hears a message describing location. The transmitters are installed in public areas, such as transit facilities.
- **Adaptive mobility devices**: Includes I-shaped bumper cane, hoop canes, PushPal, and T-bumper with wheels. May be used instead of a long cane for the visually impaired because the devices provide support across the body width and maintain contact with the ground. Particularly useful for clients with balance or gait problems. They may also be used as pre-canes. Some devices have push broom tips and others are wheeled.
- **Global positioning systems**: Built into smart phones and other devices, these systems can provide precise location.

Orthosis and Prosthesis

An **orthosis** is a device that assists the body in restoring a function. It can be a sling, brace, or splint that is added to a person's body to achieve one of the following: support, posture, immobilization, correct deformities, assist weak muscles, restore muscle function, and/or modify muscle tone. An orthosis can be simple, made of cotton (sling) or plastic, or a complex electromechanical appliance containing cantilevered joints or servomotors.

Prosthesis is a device that replaces all or part of a missing body part or replaces a body part that is no longer functioning. Prostheses vary and are individualized for looks and functionality. Prostheses include lens replacement following cataract surgery, a hip replacement, artificial arms and legs, breast implants following mastectomy, or a wig due to chemotherapy.

Augmentative Communication Devices

Augmentative communication device: An AAC, augmentative and alternative communication device, is used to assist or augment a person in communicating. The device may be as simple as a picture board containing items or activities that a person can point to or as complex as a computerized system allowing input from a keyboard, head stick or eye gaze switch that produces synthesized speech.

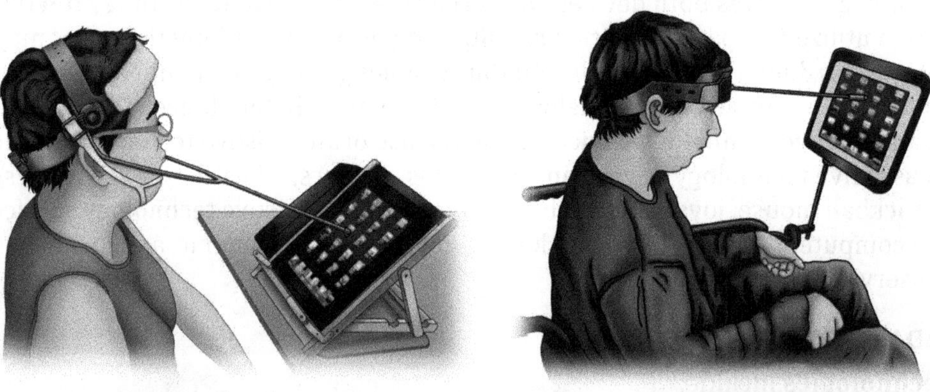

Chinwand/Chinstick　　Headwand/Headstick

Chinwand or **chinstick** is a device that is mounted to a headpiece and extends from the center of the mandible allowing a person with good head mobility, but poor upper body strength, to make selections on an input device (AAC). A similar device extending from the forehead is called a headwand or headstick.

Dial scan is a device that looks like a clock with one hand. The single hand points to pictures or symbols activating a switch that operates the item.

Vocational Aspects of Disabilities

Functional Independence Measure

The Functional Independence Measure (FIM) evaluates the patient's level of disability related to 18 items with a **7-level scale** ranging from dependence and the need for complete assistance (1) to complete independence (7), based on the actual abilities of the person. FIM items include eating, grooming, bathing, upper dressing, lower dressing, toileting, bladder, bowel, transfers (bed, chair, wheelchair), transfers (toilet), transfers (tub/shower), walk/wheelchair, stairs, comprehension, expression, social interaction, problem solving, and memory. **Admission scores** are obtained during the first three days of rehabilitation hospitalization based on observations over the entire 3-day period. **Discharge scores** are obtained on the day of discharge or the 2 preceding days except for bowel and bladder function. Bowel and bladder function scores are based on the lowest functional score within any 24-hour period during the 3 discharge evaluation days with look-back for 3 days related to level of needed assistance and 7 days for frequency of accidents. All other discharge scores must be obtained within the same 24-hour period. The FIM instrument is included in the IRF-PAI.

Job Analysis and Accommodation

Job analysis is the process by which a job is assessed and the results analyzed to determine what skills and activities are required to carry out the job, including:

- Necessary knowledge, skills, and abilities (KSAs)
- Specific work activities
- Behaviors required to complete the job
- Interactions required with others
- Type of equipment utilized
- Hours of work
- Working conditions (standing, walking, sitting, ventilation, temperature)
- Location of work

Job analysis may be carried out through questionnaires, interviews, and direct observation. Once information is gathered, then a description of the job and its specifications are developed to help to determine if **accommodations** are necessary and covered under the Americans with Disabilities Act. The 1992 Americans with Disabilities Act is civil rights legislation that provides the disabled, including those with mental impairment, access to employment and the community. Accommodations may include modifications of the work schedule, special equipment, accessibility, and job restructuring.

Life Care Planning

Life care planning involves developing a current and future plan, including costs, for individuals who are elderly and/or disabled or cognitively impaired and generally unable to manage independently. The life care plan can help to protect the individuals' interests. Information is gathered about the individuals through interviews with the individuals, family, physicians, and/or caregivers, review of medical records (health conditions, hospitalizations, medications, treatments), observations (in person, video), school and employment records, bank accounts, income, personal property, and tax records. The individuals' needs may include plans for medical testing and treatment, custodial care, coordination of care, crisis intervention, housing or facility care (assisted living, skilled nursing facility), insurance, transportation, vocational training and services. Public and/or private financial resources are assessed and included in the life care plan as is decision-making authority through the inclusion of advance directives and power of attorney.

Short vs. Long Term Disability Plans

Disability plans provide income replacement for a prescribed period of time when an individual cannot work due to illness or injury. These are wage replacement plans and lack benefits for medical services. Disability plans are often an optional benefit offered by employers or self-procured by an individual. **Short-term disability (STD)** benefits may progress into **long-term disability (LTD)** benefits or **total disability**. There are two unique provisions of LTD policies:

- OWNOCC (own occupation) refers to all functions required in the person's job. If the person can perform 4 out of 5 job tasks, they still qualify for LTD benefits and collect their full salary for a specified time ranging from 1 to 5 years.
- ANYOCC (any occupation) acknowledges a person may not be able to perform all their job tasks, but may be able to perform tasks required in other occupations. ANYOCC coverage is expensive and provides all or partial salary until a person reaches age 65.

Vocational and Rehabilitation Delivery Systems

Case Manager's in Rehabilitation After Hospitalization

The case manager's role related to a patient's rehabilitation after hospitalization includes assessment of the patient's needs prior to discharge in order to determine who will benefit from rehabilitation and establishing a plan of care that includes necessary rehabilitative services and realistic target outcomes. **Rehabilitation services** may include home health care, PT, OT, speech therapy, or specialized programs, such as cardiac rehabilitation. The case manager must obtain preauthorization for treatments and coordinate care to ensure that interventions are carried out in a timely manner and duplication of services is avoided. The case manager should review referral information and assess the patient's and patient's family and/or caregiver's learning needs and ensure they receive the education needed. The case manager must promote effective communication and intervene as necessary. The case manager should conduct cost management through purchase, agreements, and negotiation. The case manager should ensure that quality measurement and assessment of outcomes is carried out, including gathering data to support interventions.

Key Rehabilitation Concepts

- **Medical rehabilitation:** For clients with physical disabilities or impairments to restore functional ability and wellbeing as much as possible, such as for those with stroke, spinal cord injury, heart disease, neurological disease, and musculoskeletal disorders.
- **Substance use rehabilitation:** For clients with addictions to alcohol or drugs through detoxification and recovery in order to help them attain and retain sobriety and/or abstinence. Clients are assessed and individual treatment plans developed to help clients identify triggers, learn coping skills, and change negative thoughts and habits.
- **Vocational rehabilitation**: For clients with physical, developmental, behavioral, or mental disabilities to assist them to overcome barriers to employment and to learn necessary skills or modifications to allow them to integrate more fully into the world of work and society in general. Employers often work closely with vocational rehabilitation programs.

Work Hardening Programs

Work hardening programs are individualized, multidisciplinary therapy programs designed to return workers to full employment. Work hardening programs use real or work-simulated activities along with conditioning exercises and psychosocial treatments to address the patient's ability to return to work. They do not treat the underlying condition that led to the disability nor are they designed to return the patient to independent living. Once the patient is sufficiently recovered and can participate in the process, work hardening programs are suitable for patients who have a job and whose therapy can be related to their return to work; the physical, psychological and vocational deficits can be documented, and the patient must be willing to participate in the therapy.

Work Adjustment

Work adjustment training is a vocational training service provided during the period of a patient's rehabilitation. Such training can involve helping the patient to develop work habits and skills and to focus upon job retention aspects and skills. Often, work adjustment training utilizes activities designed to enhance productivity and improve punctuality. Other activities focus on the patient's ability to be supervised and the ability to work with others. Work adjustment is often necessary to aid a patient to achieve gainful employment in an integrated employment setting or environment. Work adjustment may include individual or group work, and it may also incorporate work-related functions and activities.

Transitional Employment

Transitional employment is short-term employment that is publicly subsidized and serves to join on- the-job experience with various support services to enable the patient to overcome any barriers to return to gainful employment. Some transitional employment programs are designed to meet the needs of patients with mental illness in the area of vocational rehabilitation. Other transitional employment programs may serve to assess and improve a patient's abilities in a real work environment.

Support services in transitional employment programs may include substance abuse counseling, basic child care, Food Stamps, help with transportation, Medicaid, and job coaching. Transitional jobs pay legitimate wages that are often minimum wage or higher.

Rehabilitation Delivery Systems

Rehabilitation delivery systems are how rehabilitation services and training are provided to patients with disabilities and their families at the community level. Such systems are designed to enable the disabled patient to achieve **employment** and to develop **self-sufficiency**. As rehabilitation services delivery systems evolved, the original collective consensus was that the rehabilitation service should only serve a single and specific type of disability. Currently, the concept of **independent living centers** has emerged as a new rehabilitation service delivery system. Many of these centers have established job training and employment placement areas of service. Other rehabilitation delivery systems include traditional vocational rehabilitation, occupational/physical therapy rehabilitation, and various other forms of functional rehabilitation services and delivery.

Fundamental Principles of Rehabilitation Delivery Systems

Rehabilitation delivery systems in the community usually have five basic principles:

1. The utilization of available community resources
2. The enhanced transfer of information regarding disability and the rehabilitative skills and sources available to the disabled and to their families
3. Community involvement in planning and evaluation of the delivery of rehabilitation services
4. The use of and the enhancement of referral services at the local, state, and federal levels that can create skilled evaluations and rehabilitation care plans
5. The coordination between social, health care, and educational systems

Inpatient Rehabilitation Medicare Admission Criteria

Inpatient rehabilitation is an intense program and some patients may go from acute care to a sub-acute or SNF setting first. To qualify under Medicare, the patient must meet the four (4) main **admittance criteria**:

1. Admitting diagnosis includes one of the following: amputation; arthritis; cardiac, orthopedic, or pulmonary conditions; cerebral vascular, congenital, musculoskeletal, or neurological disorders; chronic pain; diabetes mellitus; fracture; head trauma/brain injury; multiple trauma; or spinal cord injury.
2. Admission must be for a recent functional loss that the patient was able to carry out prior to the injury or illness.

3. The diagnosis by the physician must have an expectation for significant improvement in the functional deficit in a reasonable amount of time.
4. If the patient had already been in a rehabilitative program for the problem, their condition must have changed such that progress is now possible.

Inpatient Rehabilitation Facility Patient Assessment Instrument

The Inpatient Rehabilitation Facility Patient Assessment Instrument (IRF-PAI) is provided by CMS for assessing patients for the Inpatient Rehabilitation Facility Prospective Payment System to determine the rate of payment for patients admitted to rehabilitation hospitals/units as fee-for-service patients. The assessment includes the following information:

- **Identification**: Facility, name and ID/Medicare/Medicaid numbers, gender, marital status, ethnicity
- **Admission**: Date, class, transfer institution, pre-hospital living situation, and vocational category and effort
- **Payer**: Primary and secondary source
- **Medical information**: Impairment group, date of onset, and comorbidities
- **Medical needs**: Admission status (comatose, delirious), swallowing status (regular food, modified consistency, tube feeding), signs of dehydration (yes/no)
- **Function modifiers**: Bowel/bladder, transfers, distance walk/wheelchair
- **FIM instrument scoring**: Evaluates level of disability of 18 items with a 7-level scale ranging from dependence to independence
- **Discharge information**: Date, conditions, interruptions, discharge destination, discharge services, complications
- **Quality indicators**: Staging of pressure ulcers

Job Development and Placement

Job **development** is a rehabilitative service in which a patient and representative create a job development plan. This plan usually includes the target wage and hours worked, barriers present in the workplace, employer contacts, specific jobs to be developed, and any special needs of the patient with regard to the work environment. Job development activities are usually undertaken via the Division of Vocational Rehabilitation (DVR); the patient is represented as a contractor for the DVR. Job **placement** involves continued services after the patient is offered and has accepted a job. The service usually continues through job retention (90 days).

Chapter Quiz

Ready to see how well you retained what you just read? Scan the QR code to go directly to the chapter quiz interface for this study guide. If you're using a computer, simply visit the bonus page at **mometrix.com/bonus948/ccm** and click the Chapter Quizzes link.

Case Recording and Documentation

Recording

Recording results or information is essential in case management, as it provides a means to compare various programs and services to improve the quality of health care. Information needs to be reported in timely, regular intervals and shared within the structure of the system. By ensuring sharing of information within the system, effective planning and program improvement can be facilitated. When reporting information, it is quite effective to utilize a flowchart to ensure that the information makes its way to everyone involved in the process. In addition to using an information flowchart, an information mapping system may also ensure that possible gaps in the information flow are remedied.

Disease Registry Reporting

Disease registry reporting may vary from one state to another with a wide range of disease registries available. A disease registry is a database or tool that collects data about a defined patient population, such as those with heart disease. For example, a hospital may have an in-house disease registry that tracks all diseases or only specific diseases for statistical purposes. Some diseases or infections must be reported to local health departments, states, or the CDC with specific reporting requirements. Some regional health information organizations that facilitate health information exchanges have begun to collect data in computerized disease registries. Disease registries may be used to track patients as well and to issue alerts, such as when a diabetic patient is due for a hemoglobin A1c test. The case manager should be familiar with the disease registries that require reporting in the healthcare setting in which the case manager is employed.

Government Requirements for Case File Documentation

The case manager must always be aware of local and state laws for documentation that they prepare or else reimbursement for services may be withheld. The rules listed below should always be followed in particular to written records:

- Use black ink; never use pencil
- Do not use correction fluid
- Make all notes legible
- Remember confidentiality rules in identifying the client on each page; date of birth for children's records is often required
- Always put the date of the client contact
- Sign every note (no initials)
- Put the date the note was written after your signature
- End notations with the next appointment or follow up date
- Correct mistakes by drawing a line through the error and write "error" and sign or initial and date the error note
- Draw a line through any blank lines on the page (so that no information can be added later).

Ethics Related to Care Delivery and Professional Practice

ETHICAL PRINCIPLES

Ethical principles include the following:

- The patient's **autonomy** is the freedom to choose his own treatment path. Through the use of education and empowerment the patient will be self-directed.
- The case manager must exhibit **beneficence** (being kind and charitable), acting as the patient's advocate, and doing good for the patient rather than for herself, the provider, or the insurer.
- By actively seeking to prevent harm from coming to the patient, the case manager exhibits **non-malfeasance**. This is accomplished via education and counseling.
- The concept of **justice** is demonstrated by ensuring equity of treatment for one's patients. Healthcare treatment will be allocated based on individual needs. Being just or fair must balance what is best for one's patient versus what is just for the larger society.
- Adhering to the truth and establishing rapport is **veracity**. It is the obligation of the case manager to deal factually, truthfully, and accurately, establishing a trusting relationship with the patient and others.

STANDARDS OF ETHICS IN CASE MANAGEMENT

Case managers are expected to practice in an ethical manner and to adhere to the principles in the code of ethics for their professional capacity. For example, a case manager (as a nurse first) must comply with the nursing code of ethics, while a social worker must comply with the social work code of ethics. A case manager must be cognizant of and utilize the **five basic ethical principles**. A case manager must also be cognizant that the primary responsibility is to the client/patient. A case manager is also expected to conduct relationships with coworkers and other professionals in a respectful manner.

ETHICAL DILEMMAS AND ISSUES

The case manager has the obligation to act in the best interest of the patient, the payer and society at large. Clashes and conflict will occur in serving these parties, as well as by the ethical dilemma when two or more equally desirable outcomes are in conflict and only one outcome is possible. Deciding which of the equally desirable outcomes will occur is often the job of the case manager. The selection of one outcome implies that the other outcomes will not occur. The beneficiaries of the outcomes not selected will be displeased and may feel alienated or betrayed by the case manager. The case manager must acknowledge that the decision that was made was the most fair and mindful given the situation, thus reinforcing that the case manager made an ethical decision. Without this realization, the case manager will suffer self-doubt and decision paralysis.

COMMON ETHICAL DILEMMAS

Focus of advocacy is the conflict faced by the case manager between the best interests of the patient, the patient's family, the payer, and society at large. An example is a terminally ill patient in need of expensive treatment who has reached the end of their insurance coverage with a family having no financial resources and strong religious convictions regarding end-of-life options.

Supremacy of values becomes a problem when there is a clash between the values held by the case manager, the case manager's employer, the patient or their family, or the insurer. Determining whose value should reign supreme in making decisions has no right answer.

Conflict of duties occurs when a case manager, in carrying out the wishes of their client, may cause harm to others. This often occurs in maintaining the confidentiality of the patient's condition, e.g., HIV status.

Conflicts of Interest

Dual relationship is when you have a relationship with the client outside your role as case manager (e.g., family member, friend, co-worker).

Favoritism, asking a client for a favor (e.g., haircut, manicure, child care), can put you in a position where the client can request a favor in return.

Acceptance of gifts from clients should only be done under the spirit of accepting for the office (e.g., candy at a holiday).

Sexual and romantic relationships must always be avoided.

If the client's problem involves religious, moral, political, or ethical issues, **values conflict** could prohibit your ability to provide unbiased services. Recognize these value conflicts and request assistance from someone else in your office.

Ethical Issues in End-of-Life Care

Ethical issues in end-of-life care may occur due to issues involving how much care is to be rendered and what type of care is indicated in patients with a limited lifespan or advanced age. Often a conflict may develop between healthcare providers and the patient or the patient's family members as to the appropriateness of ongoing treatment or care. It is imperative that decisions to limit or terminate care be clearly identified by advanced care planning directives as to who is making the decisions.

Examples

One of the pressing ethical challenges in end-of-life care is the access to **hospice care**. Unfortunately, studies regarding access of care show that many patients in the United States are not able to receive hospice care at the end of life. This lack of access may be due to where a patient lives or to lack of awareness of available resources. End-of-life care often involves the use of drugs to alleviate pain and suffering in the terminally ill patient. Physicians are sometimes hesitant to prescribe narcotics to the terminally ill for fear of legal repercussions.

Ethical Issues in Experimental Treatments and Protocols

There are numerous ethical issues to be considered in experimental treatments and protocols. One issue is social value. **Social value** is an ethical issue in experimental treatment or protocol, which states that patients are not to be exposed to possible harm unless it is anticipated that there will be a favorable benefit of clinical, scientific, or social merit. The ethic of social value in experimental treatment hopefully will eliminate exploitation of patients.

Additional Issues to Consider

There are at least three other ethical issues to consider in experimental treatments and protocols. Such issues include favorable risk–benefit ratio, voluntary and informed consent, and selection equity.

- A **favorable risk-benefit ratio** implies minimizing the risks, enhancing the potential benefits, and that the risks incurred need to be in proportion to benefits to the patient and to society.
- Every patient enrolled in an experimental treatment or protocol has to render **voluntary and informed consent** to participate.
- Finally, there must be an **equitable system** to select patient participants. Vulnerable patients are not to be targeted, nor should only the advantaged be selected to participate.

Legal Duties vs. Ethical Duties

Legal duties are described by a society as minimum acceptable standards of conduct. Failure to perform a legal duty up to standards usually carries a punishment. Ethics are rules or standards governing the conduct of a person or members of a profession.

Ethical duties are ideal conduct for an individual or professional, as determined by the society. Ethical conduct that does not meet the standards and is not illegal is only punishable by the professional society. As a rule, ethical duties usually exceed those of legal duties. In the case of conflict between legal and ethical duties, the American Medical Association (AMA) holds that the ethical duties supersede the legal duties.

Health Care and Disability Related Legislation

HIPAA

HIPAA is the **Health Insurance Portability and Accountability Act** of 1996 and is recognized as one of the most important legislative acts impacting healthcare since the Medicare programs of 1965. HIPAA consists of five **Titles**:

Title	Purpose
Title I	Guarantees health insurance access, portability, and renewal when a person needs to change insurance plans; eliminates some preexisting condition clauses; and does not allow for discrimination based on health status.
Title II	Establishes the majority of the rules and requirements the healthcare industry must follow under HIPAA, addressing the integrity of health coverage by creating fraud and abuse controls; demanding adherence to Administrative Simplification (AS) standards, which reduces paperwork; addressing medical liability reform; and guaranteeing the security and privacy of health information.
Title III	Allows medical savings accounts and tax deductions for insurance premiums of the self-employed.
Title IV	Gives the enforcement of the HIPAA provisions to the Office of Civil Rights.
Title V	Creates revenue offset provisions.

Review Video: HIPAA
Visit mometrix.com/academy and enter code: 412009

Key Points of HIPAA Related to Case Management

Title II of HIPAA contains the rules for **protecting a client's health information**. The act covers not only formal records, but also personal notes and billing information. HIPAA covers release of **protected health information (PHI)** released, transferred, or divulged outside the agency. It was instituted due to the request from insurance companies for client information. The agency's HIPAA form must be in plain, understandable language and include the agency's privacy and confidentiality procedures. The form must include to whom the information might be released and the purpose for releasing the information. It must be signed and dated by the client and have an expiration date. Information released under HIPAA becomes protected under the confidentiality guidelines of the organization receiving the information. The agency must have a privacy officer and safeguards to protect client records. The safeguards include electronic security of files (e.g., passwords) and security of work areas and destruction of files/information.

Title II Administrative Simplification Provisions

Standardizing patient health information and financial data and use of **Electronic Data Interchange (EDI)** transactions reduce both transaction time and administrative costs. Medical providers, insurers, payers, and (to a lesser extent) employers submit enrollment forms and claims electronically and receive payments in the same manner. Security standards protect the confidentiality and integrity of all information using unique identifiers for individuals, employers, health plans and healthcare providers. Case managers must comply with the confidentiality standards by protecting the identity of their clients, their families, and the service providers. HIPAA compliance is required in use of fax, phone, and Internet communications.

Preexisting Conditions

Any diagnosed and treated medical condition within six months before the enrollment date of a health insurance policy qualifies as a **preexisting condition** and can be excluded from medical coverage under a new policy. To **exclude** a health issue from insurance coverage, the preexisting condition must have been diagnosed and either treated or have recommended treatment within 6 months prior to the enrollment date. Exclusion date begins at the start of the enrollment wait period if one applies. Exclusion of the condition cannot last more than 12 months (18 months for late enrollees) from the date of enrollment. The exclusion is reduced by the number of days of the individual's prior creditable coverage (without more than 63 days break in coverage). The following cannot be considered preexisting conditions: pregnancy, newborn or adopted children under 18, children placed for adoption who have been covered under the health plan for at least 30 days.

States' Rights Regarding HIPAA

States' rights take precedence over HIPAA if the state's laws are stricter in protecting medical records privacy. There are only several areas where states may legislate stricter requirements on health insurance providers. It is important to check with the State Insurance Commissioner's Office to obtain their modifications. States may:

- Shorten the preexisting condition six-month timeframe.
- Shorten the maximum preexisting condition time period (12 or 18 months).
- Increase the insurance break period to more than 63 days.
- Increase the 30-day enrollment period for newborns and adopted children.
- Add to the health conditions that cannot be subjected to preexisting conditions exclusions.
- Require additional special enrollment periods.
- Reduce the HMO affiliation period to less than 2 months (3 months for late enrollees).

Occupational Safety and Health Administration

OSHA, the Occupational Safety and Health Administration, was instituted to develop workplace standards and policies for industry and business to ensure the health and safety of the workers. OSHA adopts and enforces standards by regulations, by providing training in safety and health in the workplace, by outreach, and by education. Federal regulations in OSHA are directed at most of the workplaces in the private sector. OSHA has been instrumental in improving industry safety by adopting many safety regulations. Such examples include requiring guards on all moving machinery parts, broader utilizations of personal protective equipment, and establishing personal exposure limits.

Review Video: Intro to OSHA
Visit mometrix.com/academy and enter code: 913559

Bad Faith Claims

Bad faith claims often stem from the perception of inappropriate denial of benefits. Bad faith occurs when there is no reasonable basis for the denial of benefits and the insurer is aware of this, or the insurer's complicated, unnecessary, or tangled bureaucracy causes delays in approval of procedures. Case managers should always:

- Have the Medical Director issue **claims denials** that are based upon documented procedures for determining medical necessity.
- **Document** all rationale for denial of services.
- Perform a thorough **review** of medical records documenting the time, date, and findings of the review.
- Consult **legal counsel or medical experts**, if necessary, in determining benefit allowance and exclusions.
- Be aware of regulatory and contractual **turnaround times** for reviewing cases and complete within 24 hours if the timeline is not defined, and inform the subscriber if the review will take longer.
- If treatment is denied, the case manager should **inform** the subscriber of the appeals process, including the name and contact information of the appeals coordinator.

Community-Based Care Transition Programs

The Affordable Care Act's Community-based Care Transitions Program (CCTP) established 27 test model programs for transitional care intended for high-risk Medicare patients transitioning from acute care in order to better manage care and prevent readmission within the 30 days after discharge. Services include beginning transition services by 24 hours prior to discharge, adequate culturally and linguistically appropriate healthcare education for patients, timely interactions between patient and healthcare providers, patient-centered self-management support, and complete medication review and management, including patient counseling as necessary.

The ACA's **Prevention of Chronic Disease and Improving Public Health** program includes a number of provisions:

- Preventive and obesity-related services: Includes immunizations, screenings for chronic and infectious diseases, clinical and behavioral interventions, and counseling to support self-management. Obesity-related services include BMI measurement, screening, nutritional education, counseling, prescription drugs, and bariatric surgery.
- Tobacco cessation for pregnant women on Medicaid.
- Incentives for prevention of chronic disease: Test program to evaluate the use of financial and non-financial incentives for those on Medicaid to participate in prevention programs.

AMERICANS WITH DISABILITIES ACT

The Americans with Disabilities Act (ADA) defines a **disability** as a physical or mental impairment that substantially limits a person's ability in one or more major life activities whether the disability is currently exhibited or historical. However, if medication controls the disability, it cannot be covered by ADA. The FEHA legislation stated the assessment of the disability must be made without regard to treatment and the limitation needs to only make the major life activity "difficult" for the individual. Case managers should be familiar with the **World Health Organization's Disability Schedule** which assesses disability and is compatible with DSM 5. ADA protections are not extended to clinical syndromes related to illegal drug use, drinking at work or criminal pathologies such as kleptomania or pyromania.

EMPLOYMENT DISCRIMINATION PROTECTION

At companies with more than 25 employees, inquiries about medical information or requiring a physical exam cannot be done prior to an offer of employment. Denial of a job based on a physical examination can only be done if the "essential functions" of that job cannot be performed (e.g., cannot lift up to 50 pounds for an employee of a shipping company). Redress is available under **Title I and V** of the Americans with Disabilities Act of 1990 which prohibits **employment discrimination** against qualified individuals in state, local or private sector jobs. Sections 501 and 505 of the Rehabilitation Act of 1973 prohibit employment discrimination against qualified individuals in federal government employment. The Civil Rights Act of 1991 provides monetary damages in international employment discrimination.

ESSENTIAL JOB FUNCTIONS AND REASONABLE ACCOMMODATIONS

ADA employment provisions are applied only to "qualified individuals," those who have the skill, experience, education, and ability to perform essential job functions, with or without reasonable accommodation, as outlined in the job description or collective bargaining agreement. The job functions must be documented before advertising and interviewing applicants, and the functions must occupy the majority of the job's time, and they must be required of other people performing the same or similar jobs. **Reasonable accommodations** are modifications to existing facilities to make them usable or accessible to an individual with disabilities, e.g., ramp into a doorway or lowering a counter. Accommodating an individual following certain injuries or illnesses may not be possible (depression, anger, muscular or cardiovascular endurance) and will require individual analysis and documentation by the case manager. Some employers are **exempt** from the ADA, including religious or private membership organizations, the executive branch of the federal government, Native American tribes, and employers with fewer than 15 employees.

HITECH ACT

The American Recovery and Reinvestment Act (2009) (ARRA) included the Health Information Technology for Economic and Clinical Health Act (HITECH). HITECH provides incentive payments to Medicare practitioners (usually physicians) to adopt **electronic health records (EHRs)**. EHRs must be certified and meet the requirement for "meaningful use." Additionally, HITECH provides penalties in the form of reduced Medicare payments for those who do not adopt EHRs, unless exempted by hardship (such as a rural practice). Security provisions include:

- Individuals and HHS must be notified of breach in security of personal health information.
- Business partners must meet security regulations or face penalties.
- The sale/marketing of personal health information is restricted.
- Individuals must have access to electronic health information.
- Individuals must be informed of disclosures of personal health information.

HITECH also provides matching grants to institutes of higher education, funding for training for health information technology, promotes research and development of health information technology, and provides grants to the Indian Health Services for adoption of health Internet technology.

Mental Health Parity Act of 1996

Protecting individuals with mental health problems, the **MHPA** prohibits lifetime or annual dollar limits on **mental healthcare**, unless the same limits apply to medical or surgical treatment. The MHPA exempts employers with 50 or fewer employees or if requirements will result in significant hardship, specifically an increase of 1% or more in its healthcare costs. The key aspects are: 1) exclusion of chemical dependency is allowed as well as allowing separate limits for treatment of substance abuse; 2) plans can still exclude mental health treatment, but if included, they cannot have separate dollar limits from medical care; and 3) although annual or lifetime dollar limits cannot be set, the following are allowed: limited number of annual outpatient visits and annual inpatient days, per-visit fee limits; and higher deductibles and co-payments for mental health benefits than for medical and surgical treatments.

In 2008, the Mental Health Parity and Addiction Equity Act (MHPAEA) preserved the MHPA and added new protections especially regarding substance use disorders. The Affordable Care Act added to MHPAEA by requiring plans to cover mental health and substance use disorders as one of its ten essential health benefits.

Newborns' and Mothers' Health Protection Act of 1996

NMHPA was enacted to cover hospital lengths of stay following childbirth. The law applies to both private and public employers. Non-federal government and self-insured insurance plans can elect to opt out of this requirement under NMHPA. Under NMHPA, group health plans and health insurance issuers may not:

- Restrict the length of hospital stays or require advance authorization for the stays for vaginal births to less than 48 hours or less than 96 hours for delivery by cesarean section,
- Increase an individual's coinsurance related to the 48- or 96-hour hospital stay.
- Deny coverage under the insurance plan solely to avoid NMHPA.
- Provide rebates or monetary compensation to a mother to encourage her to accept less than the minimum NMHPA protections.
- Penalize in any way an attending provider who provides care to a mother or newborn under NMHPA protections.
- Provide monetary or other incentives to an attending provider in order to persuade the provider to furnish care in a manner inconsistent with the NMHPA coverage.

Pregnancy Discrimination Act

An individual cannot be discriminated against with regard to access, cost, choice, and quality of treatment in **maternity benefits** when compared with medical benefits. The enforcement is independent of the marital status of the employee. This includes health insurance benefits; short-term sick leave; disability benefits; and employment policies dealing with seniority, leave extensions, and reinstatement. The following categories of employees are eligible under the Pregnancy Discrimination Act:

- Full and part time employees
- Independent contractors
- Employees of successor corporations
- Employees of parent-subsidiary groups

Abortions and mandatory maternity leave are not covered under the Act. Private employers with fewer than fifteen employees are exempt.

Tax Equity and Fiscal Responsibility Act

TEFRA is the Tax Equity and Fiscal Responsibility Act of 1982. In order to provide incentives for cost containment, this legislation did the following:

- Diagnosis Related Groups (DRGs) determining the cost of care for selected diagnosis and placed limits on rate increases in hospital revenues.
- Exempted medical rehabilitation from DRGs maintaining it as a cost-based reimbursement system.
- Made employer group health plans for employees 65 to 69 and their spouses in that age group superior to Social Security and Medicare.
- Revised the Age Discrimination in Employment Act (ADEA) of 1967 requiring employers to offer the same health benefits to active employees aged 65 to 69 and their spouses as those offered to younger employees.
- Established Peer Review Organizations (PROs) for Medicare and Medicaid patients to ensure adequate treatment while reducing costs associated with hospital stays and also to conduct reviews of their hospital-based care to ensure quality of care and appropriateness of admissions, readmissions, and discharges.

Additional Legislation and Court Cases Impacting Case Management

The **Taft-Hartley Act** in 1947 allowed the establishment of multi-employer benefit trusts thus providing healthcare coverage for union employees who work for more than one employer. The trust is overseen by both union and employer representatives.

Wickline v. State of California found that case managers are liable for damages if their referral of patients to providers is carelessly done and the patient is harmed as a direct result of the referral. This means case managers must make sure caregivers or vendors meet standards set by various governing boards and accreditation groups.

Nazay v. Miller determined a patient must assume some responsibility for not meeting a health plan's requirements, e.g., if the plan administrator is *not* informed of the individual's hospitalization, the plan does not need to pay the full expenses incurred (payment is based on the plan's policy for covering non-approved health expenses).

Wilson v. Blue Cross of So. Calif. and Alabama and Western Medical Review re-enforced the *Wickline* decision by affirming that when an organization substantially shapes the course of patient care, they can be held liable for the quality of the care received.

McClellan v. Health Maintenance Organization of Pennsylvania held that a managed care organization could be held liable for injuries that results from a poor selection of doctors as members of the HMO network. The court reasoned that the HMO had what is called a nondelegable duty to verify the qualifications/quality of its primary care providers and only retain those that are competent. (This is similar to the responsibility of the case manager in suggesting care providers to its clients (Wickline v. California).

Linthicum v. Nationwide Life Insurance Company states that in order to obtain punitive damages against an insurance company, clear and convincing evidence must be presented that shows the insurer consciously disregarded the fact that its conduct would injure or cause a substantial risk of harm to the insured.

Drolet v. Healthsource found that the HMO (Healthsource) must act with good faith, fair dealing, loyalty, candor, and full and fair disclosure. The case also cites a conflict of interest for doctors and company personnel who 1) own Healthsource stock, 2) have involvement in key decision making about guidelines and treatment, and 3) retain the ability to terminate physicians without cause.

California Psychological Assn. v. AETNA State Care Health Plan found that an insurance carrier cannot make care decisions, e.g., limiting services, rather than allowing the recommendations of the attending healthcare professionals. The insurance carrier wanted to replace psychotherapy with limited crisis intervention. This case demonstrates the need for detailed treatment plans that support the recommended services.

Bergalis v. CIGNA Dental Health Plan spurred discussion of the problem of confidentiality when a practitioner has AIDs and the policies that need to be put into place to protect his patients.

Hughes v. Blue Cross of No. Calif. ruled that insurance companies cannot deny coverage when a physician has ordered hospitalization. If denial is done, it must be substantiated in written form and only after thorough review of all the patient's current and past medical history.

Legal and Regulatory Requirements in Case Management

Commission for Case Management Certification

According to the **Commission for Case Management Certification (CCMC)**, a certified case manager must possess the following: A current, active, and unrestricted licensure or certification in a health or human services discipline that allows the professional to conduct an assessment independently, as permitted within the scope of practice of the discipline. A certified case manager must also satisfy the necessary employment experience (12 to 24 months of acceptable case management employment experience as defined by the CCMC). The licensure or certification has to meet two **criteria**. The required criteria for the licensure or certification are based upon a postgraduate degree program and the ability to practice independently in the state in which licensure or certification is granted.

Key Elements of Legal and Regulatory Requirements of Case Management

Abandonment is the termination of a professional relationship (e.g., physician/patient) resulting in injury to the patient because there was not sufficient notice to the patient or the opportunity for the patient to arrange for alternative care or services.

Bill of Particulars is elaboration of a legal complaint providing more details and detailing more information in order to clarify the claim against the person.

Comparative Negligence is the method of measuring negligence shared among each person named in a suit, whether defense or plaintiff. Damages are reduced in proportion to the amount of negligence attributed to the complaining party.

Res ipsa loquitor is the principle of law applied to cases where proof that something took place shifts the burden of proof to the defendant who must prove that the situation was not caused by the defendant's negligence. It is implied that the defendant had exclusive control of the situation and the situation would not normally occur if the defendant's negligence had not been present. An example is leaving a surgical instrument in the patient following a surgical procedure (assuming a single surgeon was involved). Latin: The thing speaks for itself.

Agency: The principal/agent relationship between two or more persons where the principal allows the agent to act on his behalf. This is the relationship between the case manager and her employer and often results in a conflict of interest due to the case manager's obligations to her employers and the professional duties she owes her patient. The case manager, in representing her employer must use care and skill, act in good faith, stay within the limits of the agent's authority, and obey the principal by acting solely for the principal's benefit, carrying out all reasonable instructions and advancing the interests of the principal.

Corporate Negligence: This term comprises the legal grounds for managed care organizations' liability based on the corporate activities of the organization as opposed to the care-related activities of the involved healthcare providers. Examples of corporate negligence is negligent credentialing, failure to exercise reasonable care in screening and selecting providers or staff, or negligent supervision or failure to exercise reasonable oversight during the relationship with providers or staff.

Comparative negligence is when each party in a lawsuit absorbs some of the blame and thus the penalty awarded is reduced accordingly.

Vicarious liability is a legal responsibility that a person may have for the actions of someone else.

A **complaint** is the document notifying the parties and court in a legal suit what the transactions or occurrences are that will be proved during the proceedings.

Statute of limitations is the period of time in which a law suit must be started.

Examination before trial is also referred to as "discovery." This allows lawyers to review facts and documents to prepare for trial.

Hold harmless is usually part of a settlement agreement where one party agrees to pay any costs or claims. These claims would occur from the original situation.

Liability refers to the legal responsibility of someone's acts or omissions. Failure to meet the responsibility can result in a lawsuit.

Summons is a document issued to defendants following the filing of a lawsuit. The summons will state all the particulars of the lawsuit and a time limit for responding to the summons.

Subpoena is a document requiring someone to appear as a witness.

Respondeat superior: The principal is liable for the wrongful actions of his agent. A hospital can be held liable for the wrongful actions of the doctors or nurses it employs. A case manager may be held liable due to negligent actions of a provider when an ostensible agency relationship exists, e.g., the client was directed to only a single provider. Latin: Let the master answer.

Ex parte: A legal proceeding, order, injunction, etc. brought about or granted by one party and to benefit that party only, without notice to or contestation by any person adversely interested.

Fiduciary: A relationship where one person acts in another's best interest. This special relationship is usually based on trust, confidence, or responsibility and encompasses a trustee, guardian, counselor, institution, or volunteer.

Validity: The probability that the practices will lead to the projected outcomes.

Tort is from the Latin *torquere* and means injury, damage, or a wrongful act done willfully, negligently, or in situations involving strict liability committed against a person or property without the need for physical contact. **Tortfeasor** is the person who is legally accountable for the damage caused.

Due diligence is the effort made by someone to avoid harming himself or someone else. It is often used in a contract specifying someone will provide due diligence. Failure results in negligence.

Competence is the mental ability and capacity to make decisions and perform actions and tasks based upon the adequate performance of others with a similar background and training.

COBRA: The Consolidated Omnibus Reconciliation Act created COBRA as a means to allow an employee who leaves a company to continue on their company's health insurance plan for a specified period of time thus avoiding a lapse in coverage.

Indemnity refers to a traditional insurance plan where payment is made for loss or personal injury based on a contract. The contract of benefits and entitlements is paid by premiums made by an individual or company.

When the case manager makes referrals to specific providers, then under the law, the providers become an agent of the case manager, an **ostensible agency** relationship is established. Due to this relationship, negligent actions taken by the provider draw the case manager into subsequent litigation.

Negligent referral occurs when the case manager refers a patient to a healthcare provider who is known to be unqualified due to a lack of skill or judgement. The case manager must be knowledgeable about the provider's licensure, accreditation, certifications, relevant clinical experience and any history of patient complaints, malpractice, or criminal activity. The lack of skill or judgement may be due to physical or mental impairment caused by drug abuse or alcoholism, or due to general carelessness or apathy. The case manager should reference the qualifications of referred providers as opposed to their quality. Recommending several providers allows the patient to make the decision. The case manager should follow up with patients to review their experience with providers and take appropriate action to report dissatisfaction, negligence, or misconduct.

PATIENT'S BILL OF RIGHTS

The Patient's Bill of Rights was first adopted in 1973 by the American Hospital Association then revised in October 1992. Each facility produces their Patient Bill of Rights, incorporating state laws and hospital policies. It provides empowerment to the patient for making informed decisions about their medical care. It encourages patients to create an **advance directive**, such as a living will, healthcare proxy or durable power of attorney, so that if they are incapacitated their treatment wishes will be honored. The Bill of Rights states the rights the patient has for privacy and their ability to review their medical records and have information explained in common, understandable language. Hospitals must reveal their relationship with other businesses or educational institutions that could affect the care the patient will receive. The Bill of Rights also includes information on how to resolve disputes or grievances. Patients are also made aware of their role in maintaining their continued health and recovery.

FULL DISCLOSURE AND INFORMED CONSENT

A patient has the right to control the course of his own medical treatment. **Full disclosure** means presenting all of the facts needed to make a decision intelligently, within the intellectual ability of the patient or their representative. **Informed consent** must be given voluntarily. The patient must have the capacity to give consent and be an adult (or have consent given by their legal guardian). Consent must be given before a professional relationship is established and must be documented. Full disclosure for treatment or a medical intervention means the patient has received a full description along with the projected or desired outcomes of the proposed treatment, therapy, surgery, or procedure. The patient understands the likelihood of the success of the treatment and reasonably understands the risks or hazards inherent in the proposed treatment. The patient has been provided alternatives to the proposed care or treatment plan and understands the consequences of foregoing the treatment. This information must be provided by a physician with a second witness (generally a registered nurse). Informed consent is required by law and lack of full disclosure constitutes assault and battery.

MAIN ASPECTS OF INFORMED CONSENT

All clients have the right to consent to or withdraw from services. Agency policies about consent must be made clear during the intake process. Presentation of treatment or service options must include a discussion of possible side effects, risks, consequences, and benefits of treatment, medications, or procedures, including consequences or risks of stoppage of the service. The capacity of the client to make clear, competent decisions must be taken into account when providing clear and easy to understand information of what is included in the treatment, as well as alternate procedures that are available. Check for comprehension of the information by asking appropriate questions. Consent must be self-determined; it is imperative that the client has not been coerced or pressured by the agency or the provider of the service. Once information has been provided verbally and in writing, a signed **consent form** must be retained in the case management records.

Client Record Security

Agency or company policies regarding record security must be in place and regularly reviewed with staff. **Electronic records** need to be limited to those with a "need to know." This is accomplished by restricting access via passwords, an audit trail showing file access, secure placement of any equipment (computers, printers, and faxes), appropriate backup and storage procedures, encrypted files, and firewalls on networks. **Paper records** should always be secured and a reference to file number or patient codes used as opposed to use of names. Paper shredders should always be used; realize that telephone messages including names and phone numbers must be protected. Locks on doors, files, and brief cases must always be engaged. Release of information should not be done without checking for the **written client release** or **waiver**. Only explicitly requested information is communicated. Check with the security officer or legal counsel before releasing sensitive information (e.g., HIV/AIDS, substance abuse, and medical condition) Every agency or company should have a security officer designated.

Release of HIV/AIDS Patient Information

A blanket release of information form is not sufficient when dealing with HIV/AIDS information. Most states require a signed form specifically stating permission is granted to release the client's HIV status. Without specific state requirements, you are still responsible for protecting your client and should involve the client in a discussion about release of potentially harmful information. Documentation of the discussion should be part of the client's records. If written permission is not obtained in states with requirements for a form, all references to the client's HIV status must be deleted, including information about any testing and whether or not it was negative or positive.

Privileged Communication

Privileged communication protects the right of a client to withhold information in a court proceeding. Privileged communication is a legal term for a right that belongs to the client. State law specifically states the professionals who are considered recipients of privileged communications. A client **waives** their right to privileged communication if they sue the agency or if they use their condition as a defense in a legal proceeding. You must turn over certain information if so mandated by a court, or if you are acting in a court-appointed capacity (e.g., guardian or payee). Information about clients can be shared to protect clients and those connected with them from harm. These circumstances include intent to commit suicide, commit a crime, harm another person, a need to be hospitalized for a mental condition, or when a child under 16 may be the victim of a sexual or physical abuse situation.

Accreditation Organizations

The Joint Commission: Established in 1951, the Joint Commission is an independent, nonprofit organization whose purpose is to improve the quality of care provided to patients. Organizations and facilities attaining accreditation meet established quality performance standards allowing them to waive specific licensure requirements and meet certain Medicare certification requirements.

The Commission on Accreditation of Rehabilitation Facilities: Established in 1966, CARF establishes standards of quality for organizations providing rehabilitation services. CARF believes all people have the right to be treated with respect and dignity, have access to needed services to achieve optimal outcomes, and should be empowered to make informed choices. Organizations with CARF accreditation actively involve consumers in the selection and planning of services that are state-of-the-art and they focus on assisting each patient in achieving their chosen outcomes.

Board Certifications: There are 24 specialty boards recognized by the American Board of Medical Specialties and the American Medical Association that certify that physicians have met approved education and knowledge-retention requirements. Certifications are issued for specific periods of time requiring practitioners to continue their education and re-certify.

Case Management Accreditation

Phase 1

To obtain full accreditation in case management, certain requirements must be fulfilled. The process for accreditation is quite demanding and typically occurs in four phases. The **preliminary phase** is considered to be the building of an application. This phase involves filling out and completing the application forms and suppling supporting documents. After the application and supporting documentation are received, this phase usually takes several months to complete. Once the application and the supporting documentation are reviewed by the accrediting organization, the remaining three phases of the accreditation process typically will take three to six months.

Phase 2

The next phase in accreditation is considered the **desktop review**, in which the accreditation applicant's documentation is intensely studied in accordance with the accreditation standards by one or more reviewers for the accrediting organization. Such documentation often includes the following: formal procedures and policies, organizational charts, job descriptions, various contracts, samples of template letters, descriptions of current programs, and goals/plans for the departments of credentialing and quality management. The reviewers from the accrediting organization, after carefully reviewing the desktop review summary, will typically ask for more documentation to aid in the clarification of any possible or pending issues noted.

Phase 3

The third phase in the accreditation requirement process is the **on-site review**. Once the desktop review is properly finished, the accreditation review team then goes on site to undertake an on-site review to assure the standards of compliance are being met. This review team from the accrediting organization conducts interviews with management with specific emphasis upon the programs of the organization. The accreditation reviewers also physically observe the staff and their performance of duties. The review team also performs audits and review personnel and credentialing files and data. The team also carefully analyzes education and quality management programs that are in place.

Phase 4

The final phase in the accreditation process is that of **committee review**. Committee review typically involves two committees that are comprised of professionals from different healthcare areas and industry professionals chosen from or by the members of the accrediting organization. The committee review starts with a written summary of both the desktop and on-site review findings. The written summary is typically then presented to the accreditation committee for further scrutiny and evaluation. Recommendation regarding accreditation is then sent to the executive committee of the accrediting organization. After the executive committee reviews the material presented, a decision regarding accreditation is made.

Licensing/Certification

Certified Case Manager (CCM) is an **experience-based** certification, requiring a post-secondary degree in a field promoting the physical, psychosocial, or vocational well-being of individuals, that provides a license or certification to legally and independently practice that field without the supervision of another licensed professional. The license or certification must be current and active and the holder must be in good standing in the state in which they practice or by the credentialing body. In addition, applicants for CCM must satisfy one of the following:

- 12 months of acceptable, full-time, supervised case management experience documented by a Certified Case Manager.
- 24 months of acceptable, full-time case management experience (no supervision requirement).
- 12 months of acceptable full-time case management employment experience as the supervisor of employees providing *direct* case management services.

Job Description

Because CCM is an experience-based designation, the following must be part of the job description or documented by the applicant's supervisor as part of their job responsibilities:

- Performance of all six essential activities of case management.
- 5 out of 6 essential activities done directly with clients.
- Consideration of the ongoing needs of the client across a continuum of care.
- Services provided are interactive with relevant components of the client's healthcare system.
- Consideration of the broad spectrum of the client's needs.
- At least 50% of time is spent on direct case management or supervision of those providing direct case management services. This provision requires submission of both your job description and the job description of the people you supervise.

The Case Management Process

The case manager must apply their knowledge to the case management process. Defined by the CCMC in nine phases, the case management process is as follows:

1. Screening
2. Assessing
3. Stratifying risk
4. Planning
5. Implementing (care coordination)
6. Following up
7. Transitioning
8. Communicating post-transition
9. Evaluating

The case manager's knowledge must be applied across a continuum of care at a level appropriate for the client's unique needs.

Raising the Status of the Case Management Profession

Case management operates within a business community; thus, case managers need to understand the **business aspects** of their profession and contribute to the **marketing effort** of their agency/company. Case managers establish relationships with vendors and community businesses supplying goods and services to their clients; in many cases they are the only face and voice that the business connects with the agency. Case managers should present themselves as part of the solution to the nation's healthcare crisis. Submission of articles to professional journals and publications, membership in community and business groups, and interaction with healthcare leaders all contribute to elevating the status of case managers and spreading an understanding of their contributions to healthcare. Case managers should also contribute to their company/agency's effort to generate new business. The case manager has many referral contacts that should be shared with their marketing departments.

Background Requirements

Training alone does not create a good case manager. The work is complex, detailed, demanding, and challenging. Success cannot be guaranteed, but the following personal characteristics and professional achievements increase one's chances of succeeding in the field. Case management takes place in many different settings, so the **professional background** of the case manager can contribute to success. In a clinical setting, knowledge of medical procedures reduces the learning curve. Knowledge of alternative treatments and nontraditional settings is beneficial for successful case management in other settings. **Educational background** and continued education also contribute to the success of a case manager. Besides formal classes, knowledge can be gained through workshops, conferences, and reading professional journals and newsletters. A case manager needs to be credible to her clients. **Life experience** provides an understanding of how to balance empathy and efficiency, when to negotiate and when to hold fast, and when to push a client to use their own resources and when to provide support. **Personal qualities** including a sense of humor, strong work ethic, believing that you can make a difference, and a sense of objectivity are important characteristics of a case manager.

Changes in Healthcare

One of the latest trends in obtaining healthcare information is the use of electronic technologies or **e-health** and the entrance of artificial intelligence. E-health has provided patients with a plethora of information that both assists them in self-management and confuses them about care and treatment options. **Demand management** is the concept of self-care case management through education of the patient so that they can determine potential problems and seek treatment when appropriate. E-health self-care is an important component of demand management. Case managers are part of the decision trees in demand management scenarios and must make sure to fully document their interactions with patients. The concept of **24-hour managed care** coverage has received mixed reactions. Benefits include quick return-to-work time frames and economic and administrative savings through integration of the various insurance benefits available. Alternatively, the 24-hour care scenario has legal, administrative, and regulatory hurdles. Another emerging healthcare trend is the concept of **carving out** elements of a health plan to save costs. High-volume and high-cost treatments, as well as pharmaceutical, behavioral health, and vision programs are often carved out of the traditional health plan and covered by a third party.

Areas of Growth in Case Management

New solutions for healthcare challenges are sought by businesses, government, and insurers. Case managers are poised to offer solutions and services. **Public sector case management** is growing with the goal of improving the quality of care, patient outcomes and reducing costs. **Claims management** is an area that can benefit clients as well as employers. Many elderly patients need medical bill audit assistance, along with claims management. There have been cases of over-billing and duplicate billing scams that would be caught with diligent oversight/management services. Many medical diagnoses can benefit from case management. Pregnancy management, wellness programs, prenatal, pediatric, elder care, and disease-specific case management are areas of expansion for case managers. As home care becomes an option exercised more and more by patients, case management can play an important role.

Privacy and Confidentiality

One of the standards of practice in case management involves confidentiality and client privacy. A case manager must follow the local, state, and federal laws concerning the client, the client's privacy, and confidentiality rights. The case manager also must follow the policies of an employer that concern the client, the client's privacy, and confidentiality. A case manager must have current knowledge of and comply with the laws that address confidentiality, privacy, and client medical information protection. A case manager should also have documentation of a good faith effort to have the client provide written acknowledgement of the privacy policies and other notices.

Guarding Confidentiality

Clients need to grant permission for their information to be shared, whether this sharing is with colleagues, healthcare professionals, schools, or agency personnel. The agency may have a **release form** in addition to their standard HIPAA form. Anyone who has access to client information must sign a **confidentiality agreement**. Never talk about cases, even with the names omitted. Information cannot be shared as part of a teaching situation with students or interns, unless the participants have signed confidentiality agreements. Never acknowledge that someone is a client. Agencies have procedures for handling requests for information that must be followed. Review a client's request for release of information and assist those who are impaired in their decision-making capacity on what information is considered confidential. Confidentiality must be followed in the releasing of information to schools as it could prejudice future decisions about a child.

Review Video: Ethics and Confidentiality in Counseling
Visit mometrix.com/academy and enter code: 250384

Breaking Confidentiality

Confidentiality can be **broken** in the following circumstances:

- To protect others from possible harmful actions by the client. Notification of intent to harm should be provided to the other party as well as the police.
- To provide emergency services to the client, e.g., providing information to the emergency room about the medicine consumed.
- To protect clients from inflicting harm on themselves.
- To notify authorities of suspected abuse, neglect, exploitation, births, and suspicious deaths.
- To report specific diseases as required by public health laws.
- To comply with a court order or subpoena.
- To obtain payment for services. The agency would refer a client for non-payment only after reasonable attempts to collect the payment have been made and if the client has made no effort to arrange for even minimal payment.
- To obtain a professional consultation regarding how to best proceed with a case.

Risk Management

Definition of Risk Management

Yale University Hospital defines risk management as "a planned and systematic process to reduce and/or eliminate the probability that losses will occur in a specific setting and includes risk identification and loss prevention, loss reduction, and risk financing." The most successful risk management teams in the hospital setting involve people from multiple areas of different disciplines. By utilizing the expertise of people in many different departments, risk management teams can effectively identify areas of risk and format plans of action to limit or to prevent various risks inherent to the different departments.

Malpractice Risk Management

Malpractice litigation can arise from a breach of obligation: failure to do something that should be done (**omission**) or doing something that should not be done (**commission**). The person who sues (**plaintiff**) must provide two points: **negligence** on the part of the case manager and **injury** resulting from the negligence, with injury being the key to the case. Case managers should practice the following **management practices** to minimize the risk of malpractice suits:

- Utilize credentialed, reputable providers.
- Offer several choices of providers, if possible.
- Be consistent in decision making using written guidelines if possible.
- Document justification when varying from written criteria.
- Document patient discussions noting the patient's participation in the decision process.
- Document the patient's compliance in the treatment plan.
- Establish quality assurance programs to ensure consistency in decision-making and payment guidelines.
- Implement grievance procedures adhering to state guidelines for timeliness.
- Address the patient's concerns and be in contact with the patient's physician.

Malpractice Suits

To avoid a malpractice suit in dealing with patient discharge, change in treatment placement, or denial of services, case managers must aggressively seek all data necessary to make an informed decision. Case managers must balance patient needs, payers' limits (both monetary and pre-determined illness plans), and availability of facilities within the context of the best interests of the patient. The easiest way to decrease the risks involved with patient discharges is to thoroughly review the patient's medical record, discuss the intention to discharge with the patient and the treating physician, confirm the adequacy of follow-up medical care, and confirm the patient's social support network. Physicians have the primary responsibility for the welfare of the patient and cannot shift responsibility of premature discharge or denial of service to the payer without documenting their protest of the payer's decision (Wickline v. State of California). The decisions must be documented by the case manager. **Letters of denial** must contain all the information needed to appeal the decision, including explanation of the appeals process and timelines.

Prevention of Malpractice Suits

The following are ways that a case manager can avoid becoming the target of a malpractice suit:

- Be honest and open with clients, ensure clear and concise informed consent is obtained for procedures, and never promise what cannot be delivered.
- Make sure that contracts define the case manager's role as one providing help or assistance to their clients.
- Make sure fees are clearly defined in the contract.
- Abandonment is a key malpractice suit, so be sure to provide an alternative contact person when unavailable to clients (sickness or vacation).
- Maintain detailed documentation of treatment plans and up-to-date and accurate records of clients.
- Strictly comply with agency policies when at work, as well as local, state, and federal laws.
- Be involved in professional organizations to be kept up to date.
- Always obtain written consent when client information needs to be shared or when working with minors.
- Know the laws when confidential information must be communicated to other health or protective agencies.
- Always display courtesy when working with clients, and behave in an ethical manner.
- Work within the policies of the agency/company where employed.
- Find sources for consultation or supervision and use them when unsure of the actions to take in potential legal or ethical situations.
- Monitor clients and make sure they know how to evaluate their progress toward their goals.

Case Manager Self-Care and Standards of Practice

Case Manager Self-Care

Important elements of self-care, safety, and well-being include:

- **Time management**: Analyze job responsibilities, establish priorities, and avoid wasting time.
- **Safety measures**: Maintain situational awareness, ensure adequate lighting and ventilation, place smoke and carbon monoxide detectors, know exits and locations of fire alarms and fire extinguishers, establish a "safe room."
- **Workload management**: Determine what caseload is appropriate and avoid overloading. Delegate tasks when possible. Assess the time required to provide necessary services to clients and to complete other duties, such as documentation and reports.
- **Boundary setting**: Learn when to say "no" and when to recognize the need for assistance or the expertise of others.
- **Lifestyle changes**: Eat a healthy diet, avoid caffeine and nicotine, drink alcohol in moderation, maintain healthy weight, exercise regularly, and develop new interests to promote a more positive outlook.
- **Psychological care**: Maintain a reflective journal and separate from work emails and phone calls when off duty. Practice ways to reduce stress, such as by taking short vacations or breaks and utilizing relaxation techniques, such as guided imagery. Maintain close relationships with friends and family.

National Association of Social Work Standards

The NASW standards for case management include:

- **Ethics and values**: Promoting ethics and values of the profession through service, social justice, recognizing human dignity/worth and the importance of human relationships, and demonstrating integrity and competence.
- **Qualifications**: Maintaining appropriate educational requirements, licensure, and credentialing.
- **Knowledge**: Keeping current with knowledge in the field, including theory, evidence-based practice, and research, especially in the areas of human growth and development, behavioral health, physical health, family relationships, resources, and professional role.
- **Cultural/Linguistic competence**: Recognizing, understanding, and respecting diversity.
- **Assessment**: Understanding and utilizing various types of assessments and reassessments, including the use of standardized assessment tools.
- **Service planning, implementation, and monitoring**: Collaborating with clients to develop person-centered plans that meet their individual biophysical needs and goals while recognizing costs and financing.
- **Advocacy and leadership**: Advocating for clients and promoting their access to resources and services.
- **Interdisciplinary/Interorganizational collaboration**: Working with others to improve delivery of services and to help clients attain their goals.
- **Practice evaluation/improvement**: Utilizing internal and external feedback.
- **Record keeping**: Documenting appropriately and objectively.
- **Workload sustainability**: Maintaining appropriate workload to ensure quality service.
- **Professional development/competence**: Assuming responsibility for professional development.

CASE MANAGEMENT SOCIETY OF AMERICA STANDARDS

The Case Management Society of America (CMSA) publishes *Standards of Case Management Practice.* One of the focuses of the standards is on **minimizing the fragmentation of care**. Coordination of care is an essential element in minimizing fragmentation through:

- **Accountability**: Develop a quality improvement program for coordination with clear goals and a system for tracking referrals and transitions in care.
- **Support of the patient**: Ensure the team provides support to the patient during referrals and transitions in care, gather all necessary information and materials, and obtain preauthorization when needed.
- **Establishment of relationships and agreements**: Identify key providers in the community, such as behavioral health and substance abuse specialists, and their support staff, such as clerks and business managers, and establish relationships and service agreements.
- **Adequate information transfer**: Develop a system for making referrals and facilitating transitions of care that includes providing required information and establishing an effective means of communication among providers.

INCORPORATING ADHERENCE GUIDELINES OF THE CMSA

The Case Management Society of America (CMSA) publishes *Standards of Case Management Practice.* Standard F, Outcomes, requires that the case manager **maximize** the patient's health and care in a manner that assures quality case management, cost-effectiveness, and patient satisfaction. This standard is demonstrated though ongoing evaluation to determine if goals have been met and through demonstration that the goals have been met with quality care, efficiency, and cost-effectiveness. The impact of the plan of care should be measured and reported. Adherence guidelines and other standardized practice tools should be utilized to measure the patient's understanding and personal preferences related to the proposed plan of care, willingness to change behavior and to participate in change, and satisfaction with case management. In order to achieve this goal, the patient's health literacy must be assessed to determine the type and amount of education the patient requires. Interventions must have measurable outcomes and should be based on evidence-based guidelines derived from the appropriate populations.

Chapter Quiz

Ready to see how well you retained what you just read? Scan the QR code to go directly to the chapter quiz interface for this study guide. If you're using a computer, simply visit the bonus page at **mometrix.com/bonus948/ccm** and click the Chapter Quizzes link.

CCM Practice Test #1

Want to take this practice test in an online interactive format?
Check out the bonus page, which includes interactive practice questions and much more: **mometrix.com/bonus948/ccm**

1. Consistency of case management practice depends MOST on:

a. Educational preparation
b. Standard operating procedures and tools
c. Communication skills
d. Time management

2. Which of these is NOT covered according to the Balanced Budget Act of 1997?

a. Annual prostate cancer screening for patients over age 50.
b. Bone density tests for patients at risk for osteoporosis.
c. Diabetes education.
d. One Pneumovax vaccine yearly.

3. A patient with a hip and/or knee replacement qualifies for CMS admission to an inpatient rehabilitation facility (IRF) if additional criteria are met, including:

a. BMI ≥40.
b. BMI ≥50.
c. Age ≥65.
d. Age ≥75.

4. Which of the following patients is a good candidate for transport via stretcher van?

a. A patient with cerebral palsy who already has his own wheelchair.
b. A debilitated patient who is unable to sit up.
c. A patient who requires cardiac monitoring.
d. A quadriplegic with a running IV line that contains potassium.

5. Under the CMS Inpatient Rehabilitation Facility Prospective Payment System (IRF PPS), an impairment group is grouped according to:

a. The same impairment category.
b. Similar age, motor functioning, and cognitive ability.
c. The number of comorbidities.
d. The type of comorbidity.

6. In motivational interviewing, what type of talk is a client using during a discussion about improving mobility through exercise if the client states, "I'm not ready to begin any exercise program"?

a. Change talk, activation
b. Sustain talk, activation
c. Change talk, reason
d. Sustain talk, ability

7. According to the Standards of Practice for Case Managers, there are four key functions of a case manager. Which of the following is NOT one of the key functions?

a. Planner.
b. Assessor.
c. Litigator.
d. Advocate.

8. If a client has very poor coping skills and engages in destructive behavior, including substance abuse, the MOST appropriate intervention by the case manager is to:

a. Encourage the client to develop better coping skills.
b. Develop a crisis intervention plan.
c. Suggest self-help strategies.
d. Counsel the client about the self-destructive behavior.

9. The case management model in which the case manager has a therapeutic relationship with the patient is the:

a. Primary therapist model.
b. Generalist model.
c. Private case management model.
d. Interdisciplinary team model.

10. When carrying out medication reconciliation for an 82-year-old client, the CCM notes that the client's medication that is not recommended (Beers criteria) for older adults is:

a. Diphenhydramine 50 mg prn HS sleep.
b. Metoprolol 75 mg BID.
c. Allopurinol 150 mg q day.
d. Vitamin D 2000 U q day.

11. A patient who is post-amputation of a lower limb and insists he needs no physical therapy or rehabilitation is probably experiencing:

a. Self-confidence.
b. Denial.
c. Delusions.
d. Fear.

12. An assessment item that would be classified under the social domain is:

a. Residential stability
b. Health literacy
c. Mental health history
d. Provider collaboration

13. An example of a boundary violation between a case manager and a client is when the case manager:

a. Admires the client's artwork but declines the gift of a painting
b. Donates some used children's books to a client's child
c. Develops a close friendship with a client and frequently does favors for the client
d. Provides information about colleges to a client's son

14. An adult patient becomes incompetent and has no surviving relatives, no close friends, and no medical legal guardian. Which of the following should serve as surrogate(s) to make medical decisions?

a. Two physicians.
b. The case manager.
c. A social worker.
d. The medical ethics committee.

15. A nurse who suffered a back injury on the job is now attending intensive physical therapy to strengthen her core, back and upper body as a means to prepare her to return bedside and prevent further injury. This is an example of:

a. Work hardening.
b. Work modification.
c. Work rehabilitation.
d. Work conditioning.

16. The Performance Oriented Mobility Assessment (POMA) primarily assesses:

a. Time needed to stand and walk a prescribed distance.
b. Gait speed.
c. Mobility, gait, and balance under different conditions.
d. Balance.

17. The regulatory agency that oversees and monitors all health plans that provide care to Medicare and Medicaid beneficiaries is called:

a. Health Care Financing Administration (HCFA).
b. National Committee for Quality Assurance (NCQA).
c. Centers for Medicare and Medicaid Services (CMS).
d. National Association for Healthcare Quality (NAHQ).

18. The process that occurs when a person elects to stay in her home and to remain as independent as possible even though she is undergoing mental or physical decline is called:

a. A continuing care retirement community.
b. Assisted living.
c. Aging in place.
d. Respite care.

19. Which of the following is an example of hard savings?

a. Avoidance of ED visits.
b. Avoidance of medical complications.
c. Avoidance of potential hospital readmission.
d. Change to a lower level of care.

20. In a subacute facility, a stroke patient who requires 20 days of care and rehabilitation and/or nursing services four hours a day is categorized as:

a. Chronic subacute.
b. General subacute.
c. Transitional subacute.
d. Long-term transitional subacute.

21. During the interview of an inpatient client, the case manager learns that the patient resides in a low-income urban area, is divorced, and has adult children that live nearby. She is unable to drive herself and was admitted from a sheltered living facility. Which socioeconomic indicator suggests a red flag for further screening for case management?

a. Admission from sheltered living facility
b. Residence in low-income urban area
c. Divorced woman with adult children
d. Inability to drive

22. The most appropriate referral to an addiction self-help group for a person trying to independently quit smoking/nicotine is:

a. Smokers Anonymous.
b. Narcotics Anonymous.
c. Nar-Anon.
d. FreshStart.

23. As part of a wellness program, clients with average risk should begin colorectal screening at age:

a. 40.
b. 50.
c. 60.
d. 65.

24. A patient remains in the hospital for two additional days because of an inappropriate delay in discharge. These days are called:

a. Incidents.
b. Acute days.
c. Lag days.
d. Length of stay.

25. The most common surgical site of infection is:

a. Deep incision infection.
b. Organ infection.
c. Superficial incision infection.
d. Fascia infection.

26. A situation that may lead to an ethical dilemma is:

a. A case manager has a set fee for services.
b. A case manager fails to tell a client to change to a "better" physician.
c. A case manager receives a bonus payment when the client's cost of care decreases.
d. A case manager places an advertisement that lists the services that the case manager provides.

27. A patient with terminal cancer needs expensive treatment, but is at the end of insurance coverage. The family has no financial resources. The case manager is now faced with a dilemma between the best interests of the patient and the best interests of the payer. This type of conflict is called:

a. Focus of advocacy.
b. Conflict of duties.
c. Supremacy of values.
d. Justice.

28. Which of the following is a major component of essential knowledge for a case manager?

a. Healthcare reimbursement.
b. Moral character.
c. Independent practice principles.
d. Statistical analysis.

29. An insurance company has purchased insurance to protect itself from a highly expensive case. This type of insurance is called:

a. Stop loss.
b. Capitation.
c. Deferred liability.
d. Third-party liability.

30. When first meeting a client with moderate to severe dementia, an appropriate greeting is:

a. "What is your name?"
b. "How are you?"
c. "I'm so glad to meet you."
d. "Do you know why you're here?"

31. Which of the following is true about a CareMap?

a. It is another name for a clinical management guideline.
b. It is a combination of a critical pathway and a nursing care plan.
c. It does not usually include multidisciplinary action.
d. All of the above.

32. If the mother of a 4-year-old child hospitalized for cancer treatment reports that the child engages in prolonged crying and screaming when the mother leaves each evening, the child is likely:

a. Experiencing separation anxiety
b. Experiencing pain
c. Exerting control
d. Exhibiting fear

33. A case manager is part of a team of physicians who assume care for the PCP when patients are admitted to the hospital. This is known as a:

a. Skilled nursing facility.
b. Entrepreneurial setting.
c. Hospitalist team.
d. Hospice setting.

34. If an older adult is mentally alert and physically mobile with a cane despite having chronic health conditions but reports being increasingly isolated and lonely, an appropriate solution is:

a. Adult day care
b. Gym membership
c. Volunteer activities
d. Senior center programs

35. A case manager knowingly refers a patient to a provider who is unqualified to render services to the patient. This is known as a:

a. Temporary referral.
b. Dual relationship.
c. Referral by client consent.
d. Negligent referral.

36. A patient who needs help regaining independence and performing baseline activities of daily living should receive which of the following?

a. Physical therapy
b. Psychotherapy
c. Occupational therapy
d. Aromatherapy

37. A 67-year-old terminally ill patient wishes to receive comfort care measures in his home. The patient's physician recommends placement in a hospice facility so that Medicare will cover the cost of hospice care. Which of the following statements most accurately describes the Medicare hospice benefit?

a. The Medicare hospice benefit applies to patients who have a life expectancy of 12 months or less.
b. The Medicare hospice benefit does not cover the cost of medications used to treat symptoms of terminal illness.
c. The Medicare hospice benefit covers the cost of hospice services in multiple settings, including the patient's home.
d. Services provided under the Medicare hospice benefit vary from state to state.

38. Which of these is true about preexisting conditions?

a. According to HIPAA, a medical insurance company is required to waive waiting periods for preexisting conditions, provided there has been no lapse in coverage.
b. A person diagnosed with asthma 20 years ago who has not needed any medical treatment for the past 12 years is not considered to have a preexisting condition.
c. Pregnancy is considered a preexisting condition.
d. All of the above.

39. The protective strategy for insurance companies that involves limiting the maximum dollar benefits for a policy is:

a. Reinsurance.
b. Deferred liability.
c. A cap.
d. Third-party liability.

40. A client who wants to receive workers' compensation privately discloses to the case manager that he was injured when he fell off a bicycle rather than while at work. Which of the following options is the best course of action?

a. Report the information to the workers' compensation carrier.
b. Keep the information confidential.
c. Withdraw from the case.
d. Tell the patient you'll decide what to do in the next couple of days.

41. A 76-year-old female with lung cancer was placed on hospice care by her physician 6 months earlier (two 90-day periods), but she is still alive. Her family asks the case manager if the patient will be removed from hospice care. The best response is:

a. "She will be removed from hospice care until her condition worsens because she has exceeded the 6-month period."
b. "She has exhausted all of her hospice care benefits and will be removed from hospice care."
c. "She can continue with hospice care as long as the physician authorizes the care every 60 days."
d. "She can continue with hospice care if the physician continues to authorize care every 90 days."

42. If each nosocomial infection adds about 12 days to a patient's hospitalization, then a reduction of 5 infections (5 × 12 = 60) would result in a savings of 60 fewer patient infection days. This is an example of:

a. A cost-benefit analysis.
b. An efficacy study.
c. A product evaluation.
d. A cost-effective analysis.

43. All of the following are examples of community resources EXCEPT:

a. The American Cancer Society.
b. Church groups.
c. Easter Seals.
d. A managed care organization.

44. If the case manager is part of an interdisciplinary team in which two members of the team have a disagreement regarding client care, the first step to resolving the conflict is to:

a. Determine which person has the most reasonable argument.
b. Encourage the individuals to cooperate.
c. Remind the individuals that their argument is negatively impacting the team.
d. Allow both individuals to present their side of the issue.

45. A temporary partial disability is defined as:

a. Impairment that renders a worker unable to work in any capacity but carries the expectation of recovery and return to normal employment.
b. Impairment that prevents a worker from returning to his usual job but still allows him to work in some capacity until the injury is healed.
c. An impairment or injury that results in a decrease in a worker's wage-earning capacity.
d. None of the above.

46. The primary consideration in medication management for a patient with chronic kidney disease is:

a. Drug clearance.
b. Drug frequency.
c. Drug dosage.
d. Drug absorption.

47. Which of the following emphasizes achievement of outcomes in defined time frames with limited resources?

a. Variance analysis
b. Social work
c. Case management
d. Risk management

48. If a client with alcoholism expresses disagreement with the treatment plan, which includes attendance at Alcoholics Anonymous meetings, the likely result will be:

a. Nonadherence
b. Adherence
c. Adherence without progress toward goals
d. Increased conflict

49. When determining if a client has achieved a healthcare goal, such as lowered blood pressure, the case manager should:

a. Observe and measure personally.
b. Ask the client if the goal was achieved.
c. Review the client's healthcare record.
d. Consider all aspects of the client's condition.

50. The assessment tool that is used to assess the degree of brain function in clients who are postcomatose or who experienced a traumatic brain injury is the:

a. Newest Vital Sign (NVS) screening tool
b. Rancho Los Amigos Level of Cognitive Functioning Scale (LCFS)
c. Sixteen Personality Factor Questionnaire (16PF)
d. Minnesota Multiphasic Personality Inventory (MMPI-2)

51. If a caregiver has received numerous gifts from a client after mentioning that she cannot afford to continue to care for the client unless the client helps her out, this is primarily an example of:

a. Psychological abuse
b. Physical abuse
c. Financial abuse
d. Emotional abuse

52. After being admitted to a long-term care facility, a 70-year-old patient with Medicare can enroll in Medicare Part D:

a. Up to two months after moving out of the facility.
b. Any time during the stay only.
c. Up to one month before moving into the facility and up to two months after moving out.
d. Any time during the stay and up to two months after moving out of facility.

53. The Indian Health Service (IHS) provides health services to members of:

a. Any federally recognized Indian tribes or Alaska natives.
b. Federally recognized Indian tribes or Alaska natives residing in the state of the service center.
c. Specific federally recognized Indian tribes or Alaska natives.
d. Federally recognized Indian tribes or Alaska natives residing in a specified regional area.

54. Which of the following is NOT a prosthetic device?

a. Wrist brace.
b. Dentures.
c. Artificial heart.
d. Gastric band.

55. Disagreement between family members about the plan of care when a palliative care patient lacks the capacity to make treatment decisions should be managed by which of the following?

a. Pursue legal action to expedite designation of a single family member as medical decision-maker.
b. Encourage the family to consider and discuss what they believe the patient would choose if he or she were able to express his or her wishes.
c. Inform the family that palliative care planning is inappropriate unless the family can reach an agreement.
d. Encourage each family member to consider what they would choose for themselves in similar circumstances.

56. The initial enrollment period for Medicare Part D for a 45-year-old disabled patient who is newly eligible for Medicare is:

a. Three months prior to Medicare eligibility and four months after.
b. Months 21 through 27 after receiving Social Security or Railroad Retirement Board (RRB) benefits.
c. April 1 to June 30.
d. Three months prior to Medicare eligibility and seven months after.

57. A construction worker whose hand was broken on the job is being evaluated by a case manager. The case manager is assessing the client's ability to hold tools and carry various objects of various weights. Which evaluation is being performed by the case manager?

a. Pain tolerance evaluation.
b. Functional capacity evaluation.
c. Disability evaluation.
d. Evaluation by client interview.

58. The ORYX initiative:

a. Requires healthcare organizations to report performance data to the Joint Commission for accreditation.
b. Does not pertain to case management roles and responsibilities.
c. Was started by the Joint Commission in 2005.
d. Is not related to the Joint Commission.

59. When considering whether a client with a non-cancer terminal illness meets eligibility for hospice care, one criterion is that the client has a score on the Palliative Performance Scale (PPS) of:

a. ≤30%.
b. ≤50%.
c. ≤70%.
d. ≤90%.

60. A critical piece of equipment breaks down and prevents completion of a test on a client. What type of variance does this represent?

a. Operational
b. Patient
c. Laboratory
d. Imaging

61. Which of the following is NOT one of the stages of the case management process?

a. Implementation of the case management plan.
b. Medical decision making.
c. Follow-up.
d. Assessment.

62. A relationship whereby a case manager acts in a client's best interest based on trust is known as:

a. Fiduciary.
b. *Ex parte.*
c. Tort.
d. Due diligence.

63. The *primary* role of the case manager is to act as a:

a. Patient advocate.
b. Disease manager.
c. Utilization reviewer.
d. Care plan creator.

64. The most cost-effective solution for an elderly patient with mild to moderate Alzheimer's disease who can no longer stay alone while her primary caregiver works part-time outside the home is:

a. Residential care facility.
b. Adult day-care program.
c. Adult day healthcare.
d. Home health agency.

65. A patient with mild paresis of one arm is going to need an assistive device to aid with walking. Which of the following is the most appropriate type of cane for this patient?

a. C cane.
b. Functional grip cane.
c. Quad cane.
d. Hemi-walker.

66. Which model of healthcare decision making best demonstrates the principle of beneficence?

a. Patient sovereignty
b. Paternalism
c. Shared decision making
d. Maternalism

67. A patient with end-stage bone cancer has elected hospice and palliative care. The patient is experiencing severe bone pain from a tumor, and the physician orders radiotherapy to reduce the tumor's size and to reduce pain. Is this treatment acceptable under hospice care criteria?

a. No, the patient has elected to forego curative treatment, so Medicare will not pay for the radiotherapy.
b. No, the patient needs to be removed from hospice care first.
c. Yes, hospice recommends only palliative care but curative treatment is acceptable.
d. Yes, if the purpose of the treatment is to relieve pain, it is essentially palliative.

68. An infant is born at home. The mother and baby present to the hospital two hours after birth and are admitted. According to the Newborns' and Mothers' Health Protection Act (NMHPA), the length of the hospital stay is determined by starting at:

a. The time a physician initially sees the mother.
b. The time of birth of the infant.
c. The time of admission.
d. The time the patient's room is ready for occupancy.

69. The best response to a patient who insists that healthcare providers are lying about her need to transfer from acute care to a skilled nursing facility is:

a. "The staff would never lie to a patient."
b. "The doctor ordered your transfer, so you can't stay here."
c. "I'll try to answer all of your questions and explain your need for transfer."
d. "I agree with you, but Medicare won't pay for your stay here."

70. A risk stratification method that is utilized with Medicare Advantage programs is:

a. Charlson Comorbidity Measure.
b. Minnesota Tiering.
c. Hierarchical Condition Categories.
d. Elder Risk Assessment.

71. The most effective method of ensuring adherence to the care regimen is:

a. Asking the client to keep a written record.
b. Making personal observations.
c. Establishing goals and assessing outcomes.
d. Enlisting family members/friends to assist.

72. Under the Affordable Care Act, an Accountable Care Organization (ACO) is part of:

a. Mandated service delivery system.
b. Private insurance initiative.
c. Medicaid.
d. Medicare Shared Savings Program (MSSP).

73. A patient on Medicare was admitted to an inpatient facility on April 10th and discharged on April 18th. For this patient, the benefit period ends:

a. 60 days after April 18th
b. 30 days after April 18th
c. On the day of April 19th
d. 60 days after April 10th

74. When an insurance plan negotiates a specific fee for a procedure (including all charges) and pays one bill, this is referred to as:

a. Unbundling.
b. Bundling.
c. Fee-for-service.
d. Discounted fee-for-service.

75. The fraternal or religious organization that provides grants for community health projects to combat HIV/AIDS is:

a. Kiwanis.
b. Knights of Columbus.
c. Lions Club International.
d. Rotary International.

76. Which of the following is true about case management (CM) in a school setting?

a. CM deals mostly with crisis management.
b. CM is usually short term in this environment, usually only needed for a few weeks.
c. CM is a random collection of interventions.
d. CM involves meeting with patients and families on a regular basis to prevent problems.

77. If a 35-year-old client with rheumatoid arthritis has become increasingly withdrawn and socially isolated and states her family and friends don't understand what she is going through, an appropriate intervention is referral to a:

a. Support group.
b. Psychiatrist.
c. Yoga program.
d. Holistic practitioner.

78. Transitions of care are best described as:

a. Transfer of accurate patient information across different settings.
b. Care received by a patient over time and over multiple providers/settings.
c. A process of assessing a patient's needs after discharge to home or elsewhere.
d. Assessment of a patient's capacity to manage his own care needs.

79. All of the pathogenic organisms listed below are commonly associated with surgical site infections EXCEPT:

a. *Staphylococcus aureus.*
b. *Enterococcus* spp.
c. *Streptococcus pneumoniae.*
d. *Staphylococcus epidermidis.*

80. An insurance plan that supplements services not covered by Medicare is known as:

a. Medicaid.
b. Social Security Disability Insurance.
c. Medigap.
d. TRICARE.

81. All of the following are true about Medicare Select EXCEPT:

a. Medicare Select is a Medicare supplemental health insurance product.
b. Medicare Select policies are managed care plans.
c. Medicare Select plans are higher in cost than traditional Medigap plans.
d. With Medicare Select, a patient is required to use specific hospitals, clinics, and sometimes even specific physicians.

82. Case management is sometimes called:

a. Second-generation primary nursing.
b. Management nursing.
c. Care coordinator.
d. Counseling.

83. Telehealth case management services are especially advantageous for:

a. Clients with low income
b. Clients living in crowded conditions
c. Clients with poor or no English-language skills
d. Clients with access to stable Internet connectivity

84. In relation to case management, the profit or loss that results from a hospital's investment in case management is known as:

a. Length of stay.
b. Resource management outcome.
c. Measurable outcomes.
d. Return on investment.

85. A terminally ill client is exhausting all financial resources to pay medical costs. The case manager has suggested obtaining cash value on his life insurance policy prior to death. This process is known as a:

a. Nontraditional policy.
b. Supplementary policy.
c. Viatical settlement.
d. Gatekeeping.

86. If the case manager is employing evocation as part of motivational interviewing, this means that the case manager is:

a. Proposing solutions to the client.
b. Helping clients see problems in their ideas.
c. Using confrontation with the client.
d. Drawing out client's ideas for solutions to problems.

87. If, during the COVID-19 pandemic, an older client with multiple risk factors has been going out to visit friends and shopping without wearing a mask or taking safety precautions, the best approach is:

a. Repeat safety precautions at least 3 times and verify comprehension.
b. Ask the client if she understands appropriate safety precautions.
c. Tell the client she is risking her health and life.
d. Tell the client that the case manager can no longer provide services if the client persists.

88. During a concurrent review, the case manager should assess whether:

a. Care is medically necessary.
b. The client is receiving an appropriate level of care.
c. The care provided has met client's needs.
d. All healthcare providers are collaborating.

89. Which of these statements is true about hospice care?

a. Hospice care is solely for patients with terminal malignancies.
b. Hospice is for patients who have six or fewer months to live.
c. In hospice, all further medical treatment has been stopped, including palliation.
d. Hospice care is for any terminal condition.

90. If a physician in a network receives merit pay for achieving target outcomes, this is an example of:

a. Capitation
b. A kickback
c. A fee-for-service payment model
d. A pay-for-performance compensation strategy

91. If a client who has been in intensive care for 2 weeks on mechanical ventilation, was weaned, and has stabilized but has post-ICU syndrome and remains confused and extremely weak and unable to walk or carry out any ADLs, the most appropriate transfer is likely to a(n):

a. Short-term acute care hospital
b. Acute hospital bed outside ICU
c. Long-term acute care hospital
d. Skilled nursing facility

92. The organization that developed the Healthcare Effectiveness and Information Set (HEDIS), which allows consumers to compare health plans is the:

a. Centers for Medicare and Medicaid Services.
b. Agency for Healthcare Research and Quality
c. National Quality Forum.
d. National Committee for Quality Assurance.

93. Uncoordinated care that is given through multiple providers and organizations is called:

a. Patient-centered care.
b. Chronic care model.
c. Fragmented care.
d. Transitions of care.

94. If the case manager for a home health agency interviews a client who was recently discharged from the hospital and discovers that the client's electricity has been shut off because of an inability to pay the bills, the MOST appropriate response is to:

a. Refer the client to the social worker.
b. Call the electric company to negotiate.
c. Tell the client to apply for welfare assistance.
d. Suggest that the client start a GoFundMe page.

95. Under a healthcare management program for diabetics, a targeted approach to reducing complications includes:

a. Providing posters in physicians' offices.
b. Providing television commercials.
c. Participating in a community health fair.
d. Providing nutritional counseling.

96. Which of these is an eligibility criterion for CHIP?

a. Patient over age 65.
b. Low income.
c. Having supplemental insurance.
d. Outpatient coverage only.

97. When a case manager refers a client to a specific provider, what type of relationship exists between the case manager and the provider?

a. Vicarious agency.
b. Advocate.
c. Ostensible agency.
d. Fiduciary.

98. Which of the following is NOT one of the main components of clinical pathways?

a. Identified categories of care.
b. Recommendations for best practices.
c. A timeline.
d. Long-term outcome criteria.

99. The case management domain that focuses on workplace issues, disability, and job modification is called:

a. Case finding and intake.
b. Outcomes evaluation and case closure.
c. Vocational concepts and strategies.
d. Psychosocial and economic issues.

100. Which of the following is NOT an example of the handoff of a patient in the healthcare environment?

a. Transferring care of a patient from one care setting to another.
b. Transferring care from one provider to another.
c. Transferring a patient from one level of care to another.
d. Transferring a patient from one ICU room to another.

101. If the case manager is on the quality improvement committee and notes that an urgent care department often has long wait times for clients because of the time needed to contact and wait for laboratory staff for blood draws, the case manager should recommend that:

a. The lab have a phlebotomist on stand-by in the lab.
b. A phlebotomist be stationed in the urgent care.
c. The staff review the need for so many blood draws.
d. The nursing staff carry out blood draws.

102. The case management process of documenting goals, objectives, and actions to meet a client's needs is called:

a. Assessment.
b. Coordination.
c. Planning.
d. Monitoring.

103. Under the Medicare hospice benefit, respite care for relief of the patient's family caregiver refers to:

a. Inpatient hospice care for up to 5 consecutive days.
b. Home hospice care for up to 5 consecutive days.
c. Inpatient hospice care for up to 10 consecutive days.
d. Initiation of a "do not resuscitate" order.

104. According to Lewin's force field analysis of change, a driving force would be:

a. Hostility.
b. Lack of equipment.
c. Insufficient funds.
d. Competition.

105. Using the average cost of a problem and the cost of intervention to demonstrate savings is:

a. A cost-benefit analysis.
b. An efficacy study.
c. A product evaluation.
d. A cost-effective analysis.

106. A 32-year-old single mother of a 4-year-old child is being discharged after a hysterectomy for cervical cancer. She states she is very depressed because she has lost her job, cannot feed her family, and will soon be homeless. Which referral is most appropriate?

a. Food bank
b. Homeless shelter
c. Social worker
d. Mental health clinic

107. In providing care to a client, the best approach to encourage client engagement is to:

a. Inform the client about the treatment plan.
b. Provide the client with a written list of goals.
c. Conduct a client satisfaction survey regarding treatments.
d. Ask the client about his or her preferences for treatment.

108. A treatment plan that involves a patient spending at least four hours per day in a structured setting receiving psychoeducation and individual and group therapy is known as:

a. Partial hospitalization.
b. Ambulatory care.
c. A community-based setting.
d. Inpatient hospitalization.

109. If a 46-year-old male client with type 2 diabetes had been noncompliant with treatment and was switched from oral medications to insulin 3 months earlier but now claims to be compliant with diet and medications, the finding of most concern is:

a. A1c 8.5%.
b. FBS 120.
c. BMI 25.4.
d. BP 132/86.

110. A case manager is caring for a client with a chronic illness. The healthcare team strongly recommends treatment, but the patient and family oppose it. Which is the most appropriate step to take next?

a. Arrange for a second opinion.
b. Carefully review options with the patient to ensure complete understanding.
c. Consult the hospital ethics committee.
d. Transfer the patient's care to another hospital.

111. According to Martin Fishbein and Icek Ajzen's theory of reasoned action, three basic concepts include attitudes, subjective norms, and:

a. Behavioral intention
b. Behavioral beliefs
c. Environmental factors
d. Self-differentiation

112. The appropriate form of transportation for a psychiatric patient transferring from an acute care hospital to a psychiatric care facility is:

a. Private automobile.
b. Wheelchair van.
c. Basic life support ambulance.
d. Advanced life support ambulance.

113. If a 68-year-old client with renal failure and low-income states that her daughter has died of a narcotic overdose, and the client must assume care of three grandchildren but has no idea how to manage this, the most appropriate referral is to a:

a. Psychologist
b. Social worker
c. Grief counselor
d. Faith-based organization

114. Which of the following is true about a preferred provider organization (PPO)?

a. A PPO is not an insurance model.
b. PPOs offer a preferred panel of physicians.
c. PPOs use physicians as gatekeepers.
d. A PPO allows use of outside physicians and incurs a lower cost to the member.

115. The most important element when reintegrating a brain-injured patient back into the community after a stay in a rehabilitation center is:

a. A comprehensive plan.
b. Patient compliance.
c. Family support.
d. Follow-up.

116. Transitions of care generally require:

a. Change in physician.
b. Handoff/handover.
c. Facility transfer.
d. Vehicle transportation.

117. A managed care contract may have provisions that prohibit doctors from discussing treatment choices with patients if the choices are not covered by their managed care plan. This provision is an example of a(an):

a. Confidentiality provision.
b. Gag clause.
c. Ethical dilemma.
d. Clinical pathway.

118. Which of the following is the best definition of a case management dashboard?

a. A management reporting system providing executive-summary-level reports of the program.
b. A decision-making tree that provides stepwise assessments and interventions.
c. A set of tools used in risk stratification of a population.
d. A case management care plan.

119. If a client who fell and fractured a hip asks if he should limit ambulation to reduce risk of further falls, the best approach is to:

a. Discuss risks versus benefits of ambulation.
b. Advise the client to keep ambulating.
c. Advise the client to limit ambulation.
d. Advise the client to ask the physician.

120. The primary reason for stratifying risk is to:

a. Save healthcare costs for high risk individuals.
b. Better allocate the case manager's time and resources.
c. Identify red flags that indicate the need for case management services.
d. Provide preventive intervention before problems arise.

121. Which one of the following is true about the Americans with Disabilities Act (ADA)?

a. An individual need only submit evidence of impairment and diagnosis.
b. The goal of the ADA is to offer maximum chances for societal integration to individuals in both the private and public sectors.
c. All impairments are protected under the ADA.
d. The disability in question is an impairment that minimally limits activity.

122. When a patient has two (or more) health plans, the case manager should initially:

a. Determine which plan provides the best coverage and will provide the hospital with the most revenue.
b. Determine which plans provide primary and secondary (tertiary, etc.) coverage.
c. Ask the patient to choose which plan to use.
d. Assume both plans will pay for coverage.

123. Appeals for denial of urgent care must be decided by the insurance company within:

a. 72 hours.
b. 48 hours.
c. 24 hours.
d. 12 hours.

124. All of the following describe clinical pathways EXCEPT:

a. Clinical practice guidelines.
b. Multidisciplinary in nature.
c. Proactive setting of plans for a specific diagnosis.
d. A form of care coordination.

125. The type of healthcare insurance that pays in the form of predetermined payments for loss or damages rather than for healthcare services is:

a. Liability insurance.
b. No-fault auto insurance.
c. Indemnity insurance.
d. Accident and health insurance.

126. When planning care for a patient hospitalized with hyperglycemia due to poor diabetes management, the case manager focuses on the long-term needs of the patient (diabetes education, diet changes, insulin management, etc.) through a focus on providing empowerment to the patient and family to access community resources and gain education on the condition. The model of case management this case manager is using is the:

a. Clinical case management model.
b. Medical-social case management model.
c. Strengths-based case management model.
d. Intensive case management model.

127. If the organization is using the John Hopkins ACG® (Adjusted Clinical Group) system, the case manager expects that it will:

a. Decrease utilization of case management services.
b. Provide incentives to decrease the costs of care.
c. Make predictions based on the practice pattern of the clinician.
d. Help to predict clients' future health needs.

128. A physician performed a Tensilon test for myasthenia gravis on a hospitalized patient. The number 95858 was entered to bill for the procedure. This number is known as a:

a. CPT code.
b. ICD-10 code.
c. DRG code.
d. Medicare code.

129. A Medicare Advantage Plan (MAP) is a(n):

a. Supplemental (Medigap) insurance plan administered by private insurance companies.
b. Form of Medicaid for Medicare recipients.
c. Optional plan administered by Medicare.
d. Plan approved by Medicare but administered by private insurance companies.

130. As a case manager in a nurse-family partnership, an appropriate intervention includes:

a. Providing information about smoking cessation and abstinence from drugs.
b. Advising the mother to practice birth control for at least 2 years after delivery.
c. Providing vouchers for nutritious food and drinks for the mother.
d. Providing marital counseling for the couple.

131. When a patient chooses to make treatment decisions by drawing up advance directives or appointing a healthcare proxy and choosing not to be resuscitated, he is exercising the principle of:

a. Palliative care.
b. Hospice determination.
c. Developing an illness trajectory.
d. Patient self-determination.

132. A member of an office medical staff has documented a billing code for a more severe condition than the one documented in the patient's chart. This coding action is called:

a. Medical necessity.
b. Downcoding.
c. Upcoding.
d. CPT coding.

133. A formal report of a work-related injury written by the employer is a(n):

a. First report of injury (FROI).
b. Impairment rating.
c. Functional capacity examination.
d. Scheduled injury.

134. All of the following are examples of nonmedical levels of care EXCEPT:

a. Residential care facilities.
b. Adult day care.
c. Green houses.
d. Skilled nursing facilities.

135. The Patient Protection and Affordable Care Act (PPACA) is associated with all of the following except:

a. Accountable care organizations.
b. Quality reporting.
c. Chronic disease management.
d. Rewards for more expensive plans.

136. A patient's medical insurance plan includes a clause that allows the insurance plan to pay for initial treatment until payor responsibility is determined. This clause is called:

a. Coordination of benefits.
b. Right of subrogation.
c. An indemnity clause.
d. A settlement.

137. The Tuberculosis Medicaid Program is intended for:

a. Only TB patients who qualify for regular Medicaid.
b. All TB patients.
c. Uninsured or underinsured citizens or legal residents with TB.
d. Uninsured or underinsured citizens and legal or illegal residents with TB.

138. The first step in the interview process should be to:

a. Outline the interview process.
b. Explain the goal of case management.
c. Establish rapport with the client.
d. Ask the client to verify his or her health information.

139. Models that deliver coordinated, comprehensive, and accessible health and managed care from a primary care staff are known as:

a. Medical home models.
b. Alternative care models.
c. Palliative care models.
d. Cost-benefit models.

140. The purpose of stop-loss insurance is to:

a. Protect the insurance company against excessive payments.
b. Defer medical expenses until a time when funds become available.
c. Replace a part of insurance coverage and exclude certain treatments.
d. Limit the types of services covered.

141. If the case manager reviews clients' records and notes that there are numerous examples of deviations from evidence-based guidelines and tries to assess the reason, this is an example of:

a. Utilization review
b. Coordination of care
c. Risk management
d. Staff supervision

142. If an 18-year-old homeschooled client with cystic fibrosis is at her first semester away from home in college, but has been hospitalized for respiratory infections twice, gained 5 pounds, and needed a change in medications, the case manager recognizes the client most needs education from the:

a. Nutritionist.
b. Pharmacist.
c. Psychologist.
d. Pulmonologist.

143. Extensive patient and caregiver participation in interdisciplinary team discussions is important so that the:

a. Patient and caregivers can be informed of the plan of care as formulated by the medical providers.
b. Cost of hospice care is reimbursed by the patient's insurance provider.
c. Plan of care can be crafted to meet the specific needs and goals of the individual patient and family.
d. Patient and caregivers come to terms with a terminal prognosis.

144. All of the following are characteristics of subacute care EXCEPT:

a. A medically stable patient.
b. Comprehensive diagnostic work-ups.
c. Care performed in the home.
d. A relatively constant treatment plan.

145. According to the transtheoretical model of change, a client who indicates readiness to change and begins making plans is in the stage of:

a. Contemplation.
b. Action.
c. Precontemplation.
d. Preparation.

146. Upon admission to the hospital, a patient provides the case manager with a document that designates his wife to make any medical decisions on his behalf if he is deemed mentally incompetent. The case manager knows that this document is a(n):

a. Advance directive.
b. Do-not-resuscitate order.
c. Durable Power of Attorney for Health Care.
d. General power of attorney.

147. A client is medically stable but needs intermittent nursing intervention to maintain stability. The patient also needs intermittent subcutaneous injections, routine nonsterile suctioning, and a stable respiratory therapy plan. What level of care is this patient receiving?

a. Assisted living.
b. Custodial care.
c. Intermediate care.
d. Skilled nursing.

148. A primary indication that a client may benefit from case management is:

a. Six or more visits to an emergency department in the previous 12 months.
b. Two hospitalizations in the past 3 years with one in the last 6 months.
c. Two diagnoses and three medications.
d. Client under the care of an internist and a pulmonologist.

149. The criteria for being "homebound" for eligibility for home health coverage under Medicare include:

a. Leaving home under emergency circumstances only.
b. Leaving home with assistance for medical treatment or short nonmedical purposes.
c. Use of assistive device to be able to leave home for treatment or nonmedical purposes.
d. Inability to drive.

150. In cost analysis, conformance costs are:

a. Costs related to errors, failures, or defects, including duplications of service and malpractice.
b. All costs (processes, services, equipment, time, material, staff) necessary to provide products or processes without error.
c. Costs related to preventing errors, such as monitoring and evaluation.
d. Costs that are shared, such as infrastructure costs.

151. If an 87-year-old client with leukemia and renal failure has developed a severe respiratory infection but has refused mechanical ventilation, the case manager should:

a. Encourage the client to reconsider.
b. Tell the client that he will die without mechanical ventilation.
c. Remain supportive and ensure that the client receive comfort care.
d. Ask family members to intervene to convince the client.

152. If a 76-year-old stroke client with left-sided weakness is being discharged from a rehabilitation center and insists on returning home under the care of her daughter, who has had no experience in caregiving, the most helpful referral is likely:

a. Social worker.
b. Occupational therapist.
c. Caregiver support group.
d. Physical therapist.

153. Grids that outline the key events expected to occur each day during a patient's hospitalization are:

a. Critical pathways.
b. Clinical guidelines.
c. Case management grids.
d. Multidisciplinary plans.

154. Spend down is the process by which:

a. Insurance companies pay benefits.
b. Insurance companies contract with stop-loss plans.
c. People spend down funds in a health savings account.
d. People spend down assets on medical bills to qualify for Medicaid.

155. The case manager should suspect that the client most at risk for dual diagnosis is a client with:

a. Rheumatoid arthritis.
b. Bipolar disease.
c. Lung cancer.
d. Diabetes mellitus.

156. When educating a client, a technique that most optimizes engagement is:

a. Quizzing the client.
b. Having the client do teach-back.
c. Providing written materials.
d. Answering the client's questions.

157. All of the following are true about CareMaps EXCEPT:

a. MAP timelines can be in hours, days, weeks, or months.
b. Common diagnoses usually fall within a 24-hour time frame.
c. A 24-week gestation infant in the neonatal intensive care unit (NICU) usually falls into a 3- to 4-week timeline.
d. Variance time frames are also part of the MAP timeline.

158. Under which of the following conditions can a case manager refuse to see a patient?

a. If there is a conflict of interest in working with that patient
b. If providing services to that patient places the case manager in personal danger
c. A case manager cannot refuse to see a patient.
d. A and B

159. Characteristics of a skilled nursing facility (SNF) include:

a. Physicians are required to visit frequently, but not daily.
b. A full staff of sub-specialists is available.
c. Staff is ACLS-certified.
d. Respiratory therapists are available onsite around the clock.

160. The case closure domain of case management focuses on:

a. Obtaining client consent for services.
b. Utilization review.
c. Notification of termination of services to all stakeholders.
d. Evaluating the ability of a caregiver to perform necessary services.

161. The addiction self-help group that is intended for adults who grew up in a home with an alcoholic is:

a. Al-Anon.
b. Alateen.
c. Adult Children of Alcoholics.
d. Children Are People.

162. Under the 60 percent rule, the condition that requires additional clinical criteria to qualify for CMS payment for stay in an inpatient rehabilitation facility (IRF) is:

a. Stroke.
b. Amputation.
c. Brain injury.
d. Severe osteoarthritis.

163. The case manager is following the care of a patient who has suffered a spinal cord injury. The primary goal of rehabilitation for a patient who has suffered a spinal cord injury is to:

a. Promote the patient's ability to live independently.
b. Promote psychological well-being.
c. Prevent complications.
d. Educate regarding rights of the disabled.

164. Home management activities a person performs on a regular basis such as meal preparation and housework are:

a. Cognitive activities.
b. Activities of daily living (ADLs).
c. Instrumental activities of daily living (IADLs).
d. Executive functions.

165. If a client with long-term diabetes mellitus type 1 and an insulin pump has been running high FBSs and made 4 recent trips to the emergency room despite insisting that he is following the diet and proper procedures for the pump and has been using the same abdominal site, the case manager should advise the client to:

a. Rotate needle insertion sites.
b. Modify the diet.
c. Manually inject insulin.
d. Discuss increasing insulin dosage with the physician.

166. According to Principle 3 of the Code of Professional Conduct for Case Managers, in relationships with clients, the case manager should always maintain:

a. Positive interactions.
b. Confidentiality.
c. Appropriate documentation.
d. Objectivity.

167. Poverty has the greatest impact on the incidence of:

a. Hypertension.
b. Cancer.
c. High cholesterol.
d. Depression.

168. The process that protects the client and ensures that persons hired to practice case management are providing quality services by reviewing their licensure, competencies, and history of malpractice is known as:

a. Credentialing.
b. Certification.
c. Accreditation.
d. Licensing.

169. The first step in developing a healthcare management program is to:

a. Identify resources.
b. Develop strategies.
c. Define the population.
d. Determine outcomes measurement.

170. A client's entry into a case management program is determined by:

a. Interview.
b. Networking systems.
c. Referral.
d. All of the above.

171. Risk management is a subdomain of which one of the following core case management domains?

a. Psychosocial concepts and support systems.
b. Care delivery and reimbursement methods.
c. Quality and outcomes evaluation and measurement.
d. Rehabilitation concepts and strategies.

172. The difference between a Medigap plan and Medicare Select is that:

a. Medicare Select offers fewer plans.
b. Medicare Select requires use of specific providers.
c. Medicare Select offers more flexibility in choosing providers.
d. Medicare Select is usually more expensive.

173. All of the following are components of a functional capacity evaluation EXCEPT:

a. Musculoskeletal screening.
b. Review of the medical record.
c. Literacy screening.
d. Testing of physical ability.

174. When doing force field analysis to develop an outcomes management program, an example of a restraining force is:

a. Satisfaction with the status quo.
b. Desire to predict needed skill sets.
c. Need to track present and future costs.
d. Desire to use outcomes as marketing tools.

175. An insurance provider reimburses a patient based on a fixed rate per day the patient was hospitalized. This is known as:

a. Per diem reimbursement.
b. Cost-based reimbursement.
c. Capitation.
d. Fee for service.

176. A case manager is reviewing a clinical pathway for a patient hospitalized with pneumonia. Which of the following are key outcome goals for day one?

a. Check oxygen saturation and baseline mental status.
b. Start IV antibiotics in the ER or within two hours of admission.
c. Pulmonary consult and assess educational needs.
d. Administer antipyretics and pain medications as needed.

177. If a 72-year-old client with COPD was discharged from an acute hospital after a bout of pneumonia and has orders for low-dose oxygen 24 hours a day, but when the case manager telephones, the client seems unclear about when or how to use oxygen or the equipment, the most appropriate referral is to:

a. The company that supplies the oxygen.
b. An occupational therapist.
c. The pulmonologist.
d. A home health agency.

178. If a confused elderly client shows extensive bruising and flinches/appears fearful when approached by family members and the case manager suspects elder abuse, the case manager should:

a. Report possible abuse to adult protective services.
b. Confront the family members directly.
c. Notify the police.
d. Ask the client if abuse is occurring.

179. Working for the best interests of the patient despite conflicting personal values and assisting patients to have access to appropriate resources may be defined as:

a. Moral agency.
b. Advocacy.
c. Agency.
d. Collaboration.

180. If a case manager suggests a change in procedure and other staff members fail to discuss the proposed change or take any actions regarding it, this indicates:

a. Uncertainty
b. Active rejection
c. Passive rejection
d. A delay

Answer Key and Explanations for Test #1

1. B: Consistency of case management practice depends most on the use of standard operating procedures and tools. Operating procedures should be documented and followed by all staff members to ensure that all clients receive the same quality of care. Additionally, if standard operating procedures are followed, this makes it easier for other staff members to assume care of a client if this is necessary, and it provides guidelines for collaboration with other healthcare providers.

2. D: Choices A, B, and C are procedures all covered according to the Balanced Budget Act of 1997. Pneumovax is covered, but only once in a lifetime, not every year.

3. B: In order to qualify for CMS coverage of rehabilitation care in an inpatient rehabilitation hospital or rehabilitation unit of an acute care hospital for knee and/or hip replacement, the patient's conditions must meet at least one additional criterion, which includes body mass index (BMI) of ≥50 (extreme obesity), bilateral knee and/or hip surgery, or age ≥85. The classification is important because the rate of reimbursement is different for those who qualify for care in an IRF.

4. B: A debilitated patient who cannot sit for any length of time is a good candidate for stretcher van transport. Patients who require cardiac monitoring need transport in a BLS or ALS ambulance depending on the level of monitoring needed. Patients with a running IV line containing potassium need an ALS ambulance.

5. A: Under the IRF PPS, patients are classified and placed in impairment groups according to impairment categories. Then they are further grouped into case-mix groups (CMG) in which patients have similar motor functioning, age, and cognitive ability. These CMGs are further grouped into four tiers, depending on comorbidities. These groupings determine reimbursement. Adjustments may be made for short-term stays or transfers. Rates may be further adjusted according to geographic differences in wages and costs as well as numbers of low-income patients and presence of residency training programs.

6. B: The client is using sustain talk, activation if they state, "I'm not ready to begin any exercise program" during a discussion about improving mobility through exercise. Change talk expresses a willingness to change, and sustain talk expresses a desire to maintain the status quo. There are seven types of change and sustain talk statements: desire, ability, reason, need (DARN), commitment, activation, and taking steps (CAT).

7. C: The four key functions of a case manager are planner, assessor, facilitator, and advocate. A case manager must assess a situation to identify problems that need case management. The case manager must also plan long- and short-term goals in collaboration with the client, the client's family, and with other healthcare professionals. Facilitation includes coordinating and implementing the care plan, maintaining communication, and expediting care. As an advocate, the case manager ensures that the client's needs are identified and addressed.

8. B: If a client has very poor coping skills and engages in destructive behavior, including substance abuse, the most appropriate intervention by the case manager is to develop a crisis intervention plan in collaboration with family or other support systems and healthcare providers. The case manager should collaborate with healthcare providers to ensure that the client has a mental health referral and to encourage substance abuse treatment.

9. A: Primary therapist model: The case manager has a therapeutic relationship with the patient. This model generally requires advanced education in social work, psychology, or psychiatric nursing. The case manager provides therapy and also manages and coordinates patient care. Generalist model: The case manager coordinates care with different providers and maintains a relationship with the patient but does not provide direct care. Private case management model: The case manager provides individual care focusing on the needs of the patient. Interdisciplinary team model: Case management decisions may be made jointly with other team members, with different members assuming leadership, depending on patient needs.

10. A: When carrying out medication reconciliation for an 82-year-old client, the case manager notes that the client's medication that is not recommended (Beers criteria) for older adults is diphenhydramine (Benadryl®) 50 mg prn HS sleep. Because diphenhydramine may cause sleepiness and dizziness, the client is at increased risk of falls. Diphenhydramine has also been shown to cause cognitive impairment associated with its anticholinergic effects, which may also increase constipation and urinary retention.

11. B: Patients who undergo amputations often experience Kübler-Ross's five stages of grief associated with death and other losses as they try to cope with physical disability and changes in their body image. During the stage of denial, patients may believe unrealistically that they need no assistance and can return to their routine lives with no problem. Other stages include anger, bargaining, depression, and acceptance. Patients may not go through all stages or may go through the stages in no particular order.

12. A: An assessment item that would be classified under the social domain is residential stability. Other social domain items include the client's relationships, social support systems, and social vulnerability. When assessing a client's social vulnerability, the case manager should consider what risks related to work, the home environment, or relationships may occur if the case management assistance is discontinued.

13. C: An example of a boundary violation between a case manager and a client is when the case manager develops a close friendship with a client and frequently does favors for the client. This type of relationship can make objective evaluation difficult and can lead the client to have expectations that the case manager cannot or should not fulfill. Donating used books likely does not violate boundaries because there is no current cost involved, and declining a gift and providing information to a family member are acceptable.

14. A: In cases such as this one where no parent, spouse, sibling, significant other, or close friend is available to make decisions, two physicians can serve as surrogates.

15. D: Work conditioning programs restore physical capacity and endurance to enable a patient to return to work. The program is intensive and goal-oriented and works to restore muscle performance and endurance. Work hardening uses simulated work activities to restore physical and vocational functions. Work modification changes the work environment to accommodate the person's limitations. Work rehabilitation is a program of physical conditioning exercise in conjunction with simulated job activities.

16. C: POMA primarily assesses mobility, gait, and balance under different conditions. Assessment includes sitting, standing (on both legs and on one leg), pull tests, side-by-side standing, walking (including observation of missed steps), turning, and stepping over or around obstacles. Other gait assessments include gait speed in five meters with speed of <0.6 m/second predictive of functional limitations. Timed up and go (TUG) tests the ability to stand from a chair with armrests, walk three meters, and turn and sit back down. Those requiring 14 seconds are at risk for falls (Normal: 7-10 seconds).

17. C: The CMS, formerly known as the HCFA, oversees the Medicare and Medicaid programs federally and along with the states. It monitors all health plans providing care to Medicare/Medicaid beneficiaries. NCQA provides accreditation to managed care plans. NAHQ is an organization for healthcare quality management professionals. It promotes continuous quality improvement by providing educational opportunities for management-level professionals within healthcare settings.

18. C: When a person chooses to stay in her own living environment despite physical and/or mental decline, she has chosen to age in place. In assisted living, assistance is given with activities of daily living. A continuing care retirement community is an expensive housing community that provides different levels of care from independent living to full-time nursing care.

19. D: Hard savings are avoided costs that can be measured. Changing a patient to a lower level of care saves money in measurable amounts. Soft savings cannot be tangibly measured.

20. B: These correspond to general subacute. Categories of subacute patients include:

- Transitional subacute: Estimated stay of three to 30 days and rehabilitation and/or nursing services five to eight hours per day.
- General subacute: Estimated stay of 10 to 40 days and rehabilitation and/or nursing services three to five hours per day.
- Chronic subacute: Estimated stay of 60 to 90 days and rehabilitation and/or nursing services three to five hours per day.
- Long-term transitional subacute: Estimated stay of ≥25 days and rehabilitation and/or nursing services six to nine hours per day. (Patients are often transferred to long-term care facilities.)

21. A: While all of these issues may be considered, the red flag is admission from a sheltered living facility. Other red flag concerns include homelessness, poor living conditions, limited financial and insurance resources, and dependency on others for care. While reportable events (child/elder abuse, violent crime, domestic violence) automatically require full case management services, other situations must be considered individually. For example, the inability to drive may not be a problem for someone with adult children nearby or with access to public transportation, although it may prevent others from accessing care.

22. D: FreshStart is an online-based hypnotherapeutic approach to nicotine addiction, providing a book and audio track that the person can use independently to quit smoking. Smokers Anonymous is a twelve-step program intended for nicotine addicts. Twelve-step programs emphasize that the addiction is a disease over which the addict has little or no control, stressing the need to appeal to a higher power for help and to attend meetings with others. Narcotics Anonymous is a twelve-step program for narcotics addicts, and Nar-Anon is a twelve-step program for families of narcotics addicts.

23. B: As part of a wellness program, clients with average risk should begin colorectal screening at age 50. Those with increased risk, should begin screening at age 40. Increased risk factors include:

- Family history of colorectal cancer in first or second-degree relatives
- Family history of genetic syndrome (FAP, HNLPCC)
- Adenomatous polyps in first-degree relatives before age 60
- History of polyps or colorectal cancer
- History of inflammatory bowel disease

Screening may include fecal occult blood, flexible sigmoidoscopy, colonoscopy, capsule colonoscopy, and/or double contrast barium enema.

24. C: Lag days are inappropriate acute inpatient days that occur when a patient should have been discharged sooner than she actually was. Insurance companies consider these days nonacute and a form of overutilization. The company may deny payment for the portion of the hospitalization deemed inappropriate. A good case manager can help avoid the occurrence of lag days.

25. C: Surgical site infections (SSIs) are most commonly found in the superficial incision; however, infections can appear anywhere (e.g., deep incision infection, organ infection, fascia infection). They are most commonly caused by bacteria on the patient's skin. Risk factors include obesity, smoking history, underlying medical condition (e.g., diabetes), malnutrition, and a long surgical procedure. Prophylactic broad-spectrum antibiotic therapy before and after a surgical procedure can reduce the incidence of SSIs by 40-80%.

26. C: A situation that may lead to an ethical dilemma is if a case manager receives a bonus payment when the client's cost of care decreases. Although this may not always affect the case manager's decisions, it may be tempting, for example, to suggest a service that is lower cost but not as good. Having a set fee for services and placing an advertisement that lists services are ethical practices. However, if the advertisement makes inappropriate claims (e.g., "We have the best case management services available"), this is an ethical violation. A case manager should not advise clients regarding the quality of care of their physicians.

27. A: This scenario describes a common case management dilemma called focus of advocacy. Supremacy of values refers to determining whether the values of the patient, family, case manager, or insurer should take precedence. A conflict of duties exists when a case manager causes harm to others while carrying out a client's wishes.

28. A: Healthcare reimbursement is one of the major categories of knowledge necessary for a case manager, because there are many different reimbursement mechanisms available depending upon the patient's particular situation.

29. A: Stop loss, also known as reinsurance, is insurance bought by an insurance company to protect itself from highly expensive cases. There are some diagnoses that are statistically proven to be extremely expensive, such as organ transplantation and AIDS.

30. C: When first meeting a client with moderate to severe dementia, an appropriate greeting is, "I'm so glad to meet you." The case manager should avoid asking clients with dementia questions because this may confuse them more, and they often don't know how to respond or simply respond negatively. For example, if the case manager asks a client if he wants a drink of water, he may simply say "no" even if thirsty. The case manager should try to put the client at ease and provide information in clear simple sentences because their ability to process information is impaired.

31. B: A care multidisciplinary action plan (CareMap) combines nursing care plans with a critical pathway. A time should be recorded for each intervention. CareMaps expedite patient care by improving the outcome of the hospitalization.

32. C: If the mother of a 4-year-old child hospitalized for cancer treatment reports that the child engages in prolonged crying and screaming when the mother leaves, the child is likely trying to exert control in order to prolong the mother's stay. Separation anxiety is common between ages 18 months and 3 years, but after 3 years, children typically have an understanding of their parents' reaction to their cries. It is important that the parents establish a consistent routine (e.g., leaving at the same time) and keep their word (e.g., returning when promised).

33. C: Physicians who care for hospitalized patients are known as hospitalists. This eliminates the burden on the PCP so that he or she can focus on office practice. There is often at least one case manager on a hospitalist team. Entrepreneurial case managers run their own case management businesses. Hospice case managers coordinate care of dying patients and their families. A skilled nursing facility is for patients who can no longer perform self-care.

34. D: If an older adult is mentally alert and physically mobile with a cane despite having chronic health conditions but reports being increasingly isolated and lonely, an appropriate solution may be senior center programs. Typically, programs are intended for older adults who do not require supervision or assistance. Programs vary, with some open a few hours a week for meetings and recreation, such as playing bingo, playing cards, or dancing. Others are open daily and offer many programs such as educational classes (e.g., computers, languages, cooking), meals (often at a low cost), and recreational activities.

35. D: A case manager has to have knowledge of the referral provider's credentials and clinical experience. If a case manager sends a patient to an unqualified referral provider, this constitutes a negligent referral. It is important for the case manager to check in with patients afterward to assure that they had a positive experience with the provider. It is also the case manager's responsibility to report any misconduct on the part of that provider.

36. C: Occupational therapists employ motor, sensory, cognitive exercises, and various tasks to help improve a patient's performance of activities of daily living. A physical therapist helps patients with mobility and motor skills.

37. C: The Medicare hospice benefit is a federal program for Medicare-eligible patients with an estimated life expectancy of 6 months or less. Because Medicare is a federally funded program, eligibility requirements and benefits do not vary from state to state. The cost of all supplies and medications being used in relation to the terminal illness are covered under the Medicare hospice benefit. Hospice care may be provided in multiple settings, including home, outpatient, and inpatient settings. A patient need not have a do-not-resuscitate order to qualify for the Medicare hospice benefit. Patients who have activated the Medicare hospice benefit may opt to return to regular Medicare (i.e., Medicare Part A) at any time.

38. A: Medical insurance companies are required to waive the waiting period if there is no lapse in coverage. A preexisting condition is any condition for which a patient has *ever* received treatment regardless of how long it has been since the patient was last seen by a physician for the condition. According to HIPAA, pregnancy is no longer considered a preexisting condition.

39. C: The protective strategy for insurance companies that involves limiting the maximum dollar benefits for a policy is a cap. Caps may vary depending on the type of insurance. A routine accident and health benefits plan for one person may set a specific dollar maximum for that person, but a family plan may set a plan cap for the entire family and individual caps. Automobile insurance that covers bodily injury also usually has a category cap (such as $1 million for bodily injury) and per person caps (such as $250,000 per person), so one injured person cannot receive the entire amount.

40. A: Patients often disclose secrets to case managers. Case managers are obligated to report the truth and, in this case, should advise the client that they are going to notify the workers' compensation carrier.

41. C: Initially, the physician must certify that a patient who is eligible under Medicare A is terminal with a life expectancy 6 months (two 90-day periods). However, if the patient remains alive, the physician can extend coverage by authorizing continued hospice care every 60 days. The goal is to maintain the patient in the home environment with home health aides, homemakers, durable goods, pain management, case management, counseling, and social worker assistance. Routine intermittent home care must comprise 80% of total care, with in-home continuous care and in-patient hospice care available for short augmenting periods only.

42. D: A cost-effective analysis measures the effectiveness of an intervention rather than the monetary savings. For example, annually 2 million nosocomial infections result in 90,000 deaths and an estimated $6.7 billion in additional health costs. From that perspective, decreasing infections should reduce costs, but there are human savings in suffering as well, and it can be difficult to place a dollar value on that. If each infection adds about 12 days to hospitalization, then a reduction of 5 infections ($5 \times 12 = 60$) would result in a cost-effective savings of 60 fewer patient infection days.

43. D: Examples of community resources include the American Cancer Society, Easter Seals, March of Dimes, Lions Club, and others. Church groups and civic groups are also community resources. They all serve as good patient support systems.

44. D: If the case manager is part of an interdisciplinary team in which two members of the team have a disagreement regarding client care, the first step to resolving the conflict is to allow both individuals to present their side of the disagreement without bias, keeping the focus on the opinions rather than the individuals. Often, individuals just want to feel that they are heard and their views are appreciated. Then, the case manager should encourage the individual to cooperate with negotiation and compromise.

45. B: A temporary partial disability renders a worker unable to perform his usual job temporarily. While waiting to regain full function, the worker can continue to work in some capacity. Impairment that renders a worker unable to work in any capacity but carries the expectation of recovery and return to normal employment refers to temporary total disability. An impairment or injury that results in a decrease in a worker's wage-earning capacity refers to permanent partial disability.

46. A: The primary consideration for medication management for a patient with kidney disease is drug clearance. Most drugs are cleared through the liver and/or kidneys. While kidney disease may also affect absorption and metabolism, resulting in ineffective dosage, the inability of the kidneys to clear the drug may result in toxic reactions or adverse reactions. Drug dosing often must be adjusted, according to the patient's condition and glomerular filtration rate. Adjustments can include lowered doses, less frequent drug administration, or a combination of both approaches.

47. C: The question itself provides a good definition of case management: the achievement of desired outcomes within a defined time frame while limiting resources as much as possible.

48. A: If a client with alcoholism expresses disagreement with the treatment plan, which includes attendance at Alcoholics Anonymous meetings, the likely result will be nonadherence. Clients may be nonadherent for many reasons, but if they do not have a role in developing the plan and are opposed to a part of or all of the plan, there is little likelihood that the client will remain adherent.

49. A: When determining if a client has achieved a healthcare goal, such as lowered blood pressure, the case manager should observe and measure personally. While discussing outcomes with clients and reviewing records are important, the case manager should verify whenever possible because the case manager can then be sure that a goal was achieved. Additionally, if the case manager is engaged in monitoring, the client is more likely to try to comply with treatment and work toward achieving goals.

50. B: The assessment tool that is used to assess the degree of brain function in clients who are postcomatose or experienced a traumatic brain injury is the Rancho Los Amigos LCFS. The client is scored according to the level of brain function:

- No response (1 point)
- Generalized response (2 points)
- Localized response (3 points)
- Confused, agitated response (4 points)
- Confused, inappropriate nonagitated response (5 points)
- Confused, appropriate response (6 points)
- Automatic, appropriate response (7 points)

51. C: If a caregiver has received numerous gifts from a client after mentioning that she cannot afford to continue to care for the client unless the client helps her out, this is primarily an example of financial abuse. The caregiver is taking advantage of the client's need for care and fear of losing the caregiver by implicitly asking for gifts. These "gifts" represent a form of extortion.

52. D: Patients with Medicare admitted to live in a skilled nursing or long-term care facility are eligible to apply for Medicare Part D at any time during the time they are living in the facility and for two months after leaving. Patients who have lived out of the country and moved back to the U.S. may apply within two months after returning to the U.S. Patients who move out of their prescription drug plan's service area can change plans beginning a month prior to the move and up to two months after the move.

53. A: The Indian Health Service, a division of HHS, provides health services to members of any federally recognized Indian tribes and Alaska natives directly or through contracted service. If IHS provides service through a specific tribal contract, in that case, services are provided first to tribal members and then to members of other tribes/Alaskan natives as space allows. There are currently 33 IHS hospitals, 50 health stations, and 59 IHS health centers, but the availability of IHS health services is not adequate to meet needs, especially outside of reservation areas.

54. A: Prosthetic devices are artificial replacements for a part of the body that is missing due to birth defect or injury. Prosthetic devices can also be placed inside the body, such as an artificial heart, dentures, artificial lungs, or a gastric band. A wrist brace is an orthotic device. Orthotics are applied externally to a part of the body to support, align, or improve movement.

55. B: When terminally ill patients lack the mental capacity to make end-of-life treatment decisions, family members usually become the primary medical decision-makers in the absence of a predetermined health care power of attorney. Family members may have conflicting values and opinions about end-of-life issues. Convening a family conference with palliative care providers is helpful in cases where there is disagreement among family members regarding the plan of care. Once the family members are updated about the medical status of the patient, a respectful and honest conversation should take place in which each family member's opinions and concerns about what the plan of care should be are elicited. Members of the palliative care team can encourage family members to consider what they believe the patient would have wanted if he or she were able to decide for himself or herself. This may be quite different from what they would choose for themselves in a similar situation.

56. B: Patients who are under 65 and newly disabled may apply for Medicare, with coverage beginning 24 months after the person begins getting SS or RRB disability benefits; however, the patient can apply for Medicare Part D between months 21 and 27 after receiving SS or RRB benefits, so patients should be advised to apply at month 21 to avoid delay in receiving Medicare Part D benefits. Patients who are already eligible because of disability and turn 65 can enroll for Medicare Part D during the period extending from three months prior to turning 65 to three months after.

57. B: The functional capacity exam is a process of assessing a person's physical and functional abilities to perform tasks. In order to assess this particular client, he will need to be able to use his hand to safely use tools and move objects, therefore these abilities must be assessed prior to the client returning to work. The patient's performance level should match the demands of the occupation in question. The purpose of the exam is to determine if a patient is ready to go back to work after an injury.

58. A: ORYX (Outcome Research Yields Excellence) requires hospitals to collect data and transmit them to the Joint Commission for a minimum of four core measure sets to evaluate the performance data for accreditation purposes. The initiative was started by the Joint Commission in 1997. Case managers who work in Joint-Commission-accredited organizations should understand the importance of case manager roles and responsibilities because they are crucial to accreditation.

59. B: When considering whether a client with a non-cancer terminal illness meets eligibility for hospice care, one criterion is that the client has a score on the Palliative Performance Scale (PPS) of ≤50% with declining function. For a client with terminal cancer, the score may be ≤70%. Other criteria include the expectation of death within 6 months, dependence in 3 or more activities of daily living, altered body weight (>10% loss of weight over previous 4 to 6 months), and deterioration in overall condition over the previous 4 to 6 months (more hospitalizations or ED visits, decreased physical activity, impaired cognition).

60. A: A variance is anything that does not happen how and when it is supposed to happen. If a piece of equipment breaks down before patient testing is complete, an operational variance has occurred. In the case of healthcare professional variances, the provider causes a delay in attaining the expected outcome. Patient variances may cause delays due to unexpected changes in patient condition or due to refusal of a procedure.

61. B: Case managers do not make medical decisions. That is the domain of the physician. Stages of the case management process include implementation of the case management plan, follow-up, assessment, problem identification, coordination of the case plan, and continuous monitoring and reevaluation.

62. A: A case manager establishes a relationship with a client to advocate for his best interests. This makes the case manager a fiduciary. The term *ex parte* refers to a legal proceeding or a legal order.

A tort, on the other hand, refers to a wrongful act performed willfully. When a person investigates a business or personal relationship prior to signing a contract, he is performing due diligence.

63. A: Patient advocate is the best answer. Advocacy is essential to a case manager's daily practice. A case manager acts on behalf of clients who may not be able to speak for themselves or who are not knowledgeable about health care. Above all, the case manager should always have the client's best interest in mind.

64. B: An adult day-care program designed for Alzheimer's patients is the most cost-effective solution. These programs vary, but average about $65 per day, and some are supported by grants to defray costs for those with low income. Adult day healthcare programs are health-focused programs with RNs and therapists (speech, physical, occupational) available with costs depending on services utilized. Residential care facilities may cost from $2,000 to $8,000 or more monthly. Home Health Agencies charge on an hourly basis, usually about $25 per hour for an aide.

65. C: The quad cane would be most appropriate for this patient. It has a rectangular base with four supports that contact the walking surface. These are more appropriate for patients who need more balance assistance, such as those with mild paresis of an arm or a mild hemiparesis. The simplest cane is the C cane, a straight cane with a curved handle for those who need slight assistance. A functional grip cane has a straight rather than curved handle and allows for an improved grip and more support than C canes. Hemi-walkers have a much larger base than a quad cane and provide more support for patients with more severe hemiplegia.

66. B: A relationship between healthcare practitioners and patients is paternalistic and beneficent. This means that people trust the practitioner to do what is in the best medical interest of the patient. Paternalism is justified in that patients usually don't comprehend medical concepts well enough to make the correct decision about their care. In the patient sovereignty model, the patient is "boss." In this case, one could argue that the patient knows better than anyone else what is in his best interests. Shared decision making means the healthcare team and the patient work together.

67. D: Palliative care provides comfort rather than curative treatment, although curative treatment may also relieve pain or symptoms. Thus, there is no clear line between the two. Palliative care is meant to improve the quality of life and to relieve suffering, but it does not include treatments solely intended to prolong life or hasten death. The goals of palliative care are to provide adequate pain management and relief of symptoms (such as nausea or shortness of breath), to provide support for both the patient and caregivers or family, and to ensure that patients and family receive psychosocial, spiritual, and bereavement support.

68. C: According to the NMHPA, the length of hospital stay is determined by starting at the time of admission if delivery occurs outside the hospital. If delivery occurs in the hospital, it begins at the time of delivery. In the case of multiple births, it begins at the time the last infant is born.

69. C: The best response to a patient who believes the staff is lying is to state, "I'll try to answer all of your questions and explain your need for transfer." The case manager should avoid agreeing or disagreeing as this suggests the case manager is in a position to pass judgment. The case manager should not attempt to defend the doctor or the system because this may make the patient feel the case manager is taking sides. The case manager should calmly allow the patient to vent and answer questions and provide information.

70. C: The Hierarchical Condition Categories is a risk stratification utilized by CMS as part of the Medicare Advantage program, based on ICD-10 diagnostic codes for 70 condition categories, to estimate the costs of care for the year. A risk adjustment factor (numeric risk score) is applied to each diagnostic code, and the total then is utilized to determine appropriate estimated costs for care. HCC is increasingly used by other insurance companies as well to estimate cost.

71. C: The most effective method of ensuring adherence to the care regimen is establishing goals and assessing outcomes. The goals should be developed in cooperation with the client and/or family/caregiver so the person has a sense of ownership and clearly understands the measures that will determine compliance. The goals and outcomes should be assessed regularly and feedback provided to the client and/or family/caregiver about progress toward meeting goals and modifications made when indicated.

72. D: Under the Affordable Care Act, an Accountable Care Organization (ACO) is part of Medicare Shared Savings Program (MSSP), in which volunteer groups of physicians and other healthcare providers and medical facilities form an organization to provide and coordinate care to groups of beneficiaries (minimum 5,000) in return for financial incentives. The ACO must participate for a minimum of three years and must institute quality measures and cost-containment strategies. The ACO receives a percentage of savings based on benchmark levels.

73. A: With Medicare, the benefit period, which began on admission to an inpatient facility, ends after the patient has been out of a medical facility for 60 days (including the day of discharge). Patients can have multiple benefit periods in one year but have to pay a hospital deductible for each benefit period. The first 60 days require no coinsurance but from days 61 to 90, the patient must pay a daily coinsurance charge. Hospitalization over 90 days requires use of lifetime reserve (for up to 60 days) or other form of payment.

74. B: Bundling occurs when an insurance plan negotiates a specific fee for a procedure, including all associated costs, and pays one bill. Unbundling occurs when a bundled agreement is dissolved, and the insurance plan pays separate bills (hospital, anesthesiologist, surgeon, etc.). Fee-for-service is the traditional billing method in which services are billed separately. Discounted fee-for-service is similar to fee-for-service except that reimbursements are discounted.

75. D: Rotary International focuses on six areas for grants, including two that focus on health: disease prevention and treatment (which provides grants to combat the spread of HIV/AIDS) and maternal and child health. Kiwanis provides grants to clubs to support projects that serve children. The Knights of Columbus provides funding for many charitable endeavors, including a focus on the needs of people with physical/developmental disabilities and support of the Special Olympics. Lions Club International contributes to many causes and focuses on initiatives for vision screening, prevention of blindness, and disabilities, including diabetes prevention and treatment.

76. D: Case management in the school is a long-term relationship with a child and his family, usually lasting throughout the academic year. It includes comprehensive involvement and coordination of services to meet a child's healthcare needs. It is far more than crisis and problem management. Interventions are organized and not random. The goal of case management in schools is to decrease fragmented care and to improve the quality of life for children with chronic illnesses.

77. A: If a 35-year-old client with rheumatoid arthritis has become increasingly withdrawn and socially isolated and states that her family and friends don't understand what she is going through, an appropriate intervention is referral to a support group. Clients with chronic illnesses often benefit from participating in a support group with others with the same disease because clients often find that they can express what they are feeling and the challenges they face more freely and gain insight from the group regarding coping strategies.

78. A: Transitions of care involve transfer of accurate patient information across different settings. Transfer from a rehabilitation facility to a skilled nursing facility is an example of a care transfer. Having good transitional care plans in place minimizes the risk of adverse events during transfer. Care received by a patient over time and over multiple providers/settings describes continuity of care. A process of assessing a patient's needs after discharge to home or elsewhere refers to discharge planning. Assessment of a patient's capacity to manage his own care needs defines functional status.

79. C: Surgical site infections are most commonly caused by *Staphylococcus aureus, Enterococcus* spp., and *Staphylococcus epidermidis. Streptococcus pneumoniae* is a common cause of pneumonia.

80. C: Medigap plans are insurance plans that supplement services not covered by Medicare. On the other hand, Medicaid is federally funded insurance for the poor. TRICARE is related to military.

81. C: Medicare Select plans have lower premiums than Medigap policies because of their requirement to use specific facilities and, sometimes, specific physicians. All of the other statements are true.

82. A: Nursing case management is an offshoot of primary nursing. It allows for care focused on outcomes within a cost-containment framework. Case management and care coordination are often used interchangeably but are in fact, different. Care coordination focuses on coordinating the parties involved in the patient's care, while case management is service-focused. Counseling involves therapy while case management is focused on coordinating any and all services required to rehabilitate the patient without providing therapy directly.

83. D: Telehealth case management services are especially advantageous for clients with stable Internet connectivity, assuming that they are computer literate. However, telehealthcare may result in barriers for some clients, such as those with low income who may live in crowded conditions lacking privacy or who may lack Internet connectivity. Some clients lack basic computer skills that allow them to maneuver through a site and to connect. Clients with poor or no English-language skills may have difficulty comprehending communication.

84. D: Return on investment (ROI) is the profit or loss that results from a hospital's investment in case management. To calculate ROI, compare costs of case management resources versus the benefits it produces by using the formula:

$$\frac{\text{benefits} - \text{costs}}{\text{costs}} \times 100\% = \%\ \text{ROI}$$

85. C: This scenario describes the process known as a viatical settlement whereby a patient can obtain cash value from a life insurance policy prior to death.

86. D: If the case manager is employing evocation as part of motivational interviewing, this means that the case manager is drawing out client's ideas for solutions to problems. Motivational interviewing focuses on the role of motivation in eliciting change and identifies individualized strategies.

- Elements: Collaboration, evocation, autonomy.
- Principles: Expression of empathy, support of self-efficacy, acceptance of resistance, and examination of discrepancies.
- Strategies: Avoiding yes/no questions, providing affirmations, providing reflective listening, providing summaries, and encouraging change talk.

87. A: If during the COVID-19 pandemic, an older client with multiple risk factors has been going out to visit friends and shopping without wearing a mask or taking safety precautions, the best approach is to repeat safety precaution at least 3 times—in different words—and to verify comprehension. Older clients, especially, may benefit from repetition; however, even with comprehension, some clients will do as they please, and the case manager may have little control over that.

88. B: A concurrent review is generally carried out when a client is hospitalized in order to determine if the client is receiving an appropriate level of care. The case manager should interview the client and review the client's history and medical records. The concurrent review is utilized to determine whether or not a client needs to remain hospitalized or could be discharged or transferred to another level of care, such as to a subacute facility or skilled nursing facility.

89. D: Hospice care being solely for patients with terminal malignancies or that hospice care requires the cessation of medical and palliative care are common misconceptions. Hospice is for patients with any terminal condition. Life expectancy has no bearing on hospice care. Even in the face of discontinuing aggressive therapy, patients in hospice care should receive palliative care to maximize comfort.

90. D: If a physician in a network receives merit pay for achieving target outcomes, this is an example of a pay-for-performance compensation strategy. In this case, the network would provide guidelines explaining how the physician qualifies to receive the bonus payment and how frequently, such as quarterly or annually. One advantage of the pay-for-performance system is that the physician's salary is not capped, encouraging him or her to participate. Additionally, because targets are usually cost-saving measures, the pay-for-performance payments do not generally reflect added costs to the organization.

91. C: If a client who has been in intensive care for 2 weeks on mechanical ventilation, was weaned, and has stabilized but has post-ICU syndrome and remains confused and extremely weak and unable to walk or carry out any ADLs, the most appropriate transfer is likely to a long-term acute care hospital (AKA post-ICU care). Post-ICU syndrome may persist for weeks or months, and in some cases some deficits will remain permanently.

92. D: The National Committee for Quality Assurance (NCQA) developed the Healthcare Effectiveness and Information Set (HEDIS) as performance measures that allow consumers to compare health plans. Most health plans collect and report HEDIS data, and Medicare requires HEDIS data for HMOs. NCQA's goal is to improve the quality of healthcare through the use of evidence-based research and works with many agencies at the state and federal level to develop healthcare policies.

93. C: Fragmented care occurs when uncoordinated care is given via multiple clinicians and organizations. It is a widely recognized problem. Efforts are now focusing on improving communication among healthcare providers in situations such as when a patient is discharged from the hospital. Patient-centered care involves treating patients as partners in health care, urging them to take responsibility for their health, and involving them in planning. Chronic care models are models for assessment and treatment of chronically ill patients.

94. A: If the case manager for a home health agency interviews a client who was recently discharged from the hospital and discovers that the client's electricity has been shut off because of an inability to pay the bills, the most appropriate response is to refer the client to the social worker.

Assessing the client's financial status and determining eligibility for public assistance is the responsibility of a social worker, who has the training needed to effectively deal with these issues.

95. D: In a targeted approach, healthcare management focuses on the needs of a specific patient or a group of patients with similar problems. In this case, providing nutritional counseling directly to patients who are not adequately controlling their diabetes may improve outcomes by preventing complications and frequent hospitalizations and may reduce costs. These programs may set individual target goals as well, such as a specific weight loss or maintenance of a specific range for blood glucose levels.

96. B: The *Children's Health Insurance Program (CHIP) is an insurance* program for children. To be eligible for CHIP, federal guidelines must be met. The child's family must be of low-income status, not qualify for Medicaid, and not have any medical insurance. CHIP does cover inpatient services in addition to outpatient services.

97. C: The relationship that exists between the case manager and a referral provider is an ostensible agency. If that provider were to perform negligent actions, the referring case manager may also become subject to litigation. A fiduciary is a relationship whereby the case manager acts in the client's best interests. The case manager is an advocate for the client, not the provider.

98. B: There are four main components of clinical pathways: identified categories of care, a timeline, outcome criteria, and allowance for variances.

99. C: The vocational concepts and strategies domain is a case management domain concentration on disability issues, identifying accessibility barriers in the client's home, determining the need for rehabilitative services, and arranging vocational services.

100. D: Handoffs involve three types of transfers: from one provider to another, one setting to another, and from one level of care to another. Occasionally, patient's rooms change within the same hospital unit, but the providers, level of care, and setting remain the same otherwise. In this case a handoff is not performed.

101. B: If the case manager is on the quality improvement committee and notes that an urgent care department often has long wait times for clients because of the time needed to contact and wait for laboratory staff for blood draws, the case manager should recommend that a phlebotomist be stationed in the urgent care. Blood draws are common in urgent care, but nursing staff are frequently already overburdened. Reducing wait time will increase the rate of client turnover and increase overall efficiency.

102. C: Planning is the process by which a case manager documents goals, objectives, and actions that will meet a client's needs. Assessment entails gathering data about a client's special needs and situation prior to forming a case management plan. Coordination involves organization, modification, and documentation of resources necessary to achieve goals set forth in the plan, and monitoring involves securing information needed to gauge the effectiveness of the plan.

103. A: The Medicare hospice benefit is a federal program for Medicare-eligible patients with an estimated life expectancy of 6 months or less. The cost of all supplies and medications being used in relation to the terminal illness are covered. The Medicare hospice benefit covers inpatient respite care for up to 5 consecutive days to provide short-term relief to a hospice patient's primary caregiver. Additionally, the Medicare hospice benefit covers routine home care, inpatient care for medical conditions or complications related to the terminal illness, and continuous home care for medical complications that would otherwise require inpatient hospitalization.

104. D: According to Lewin's force field analysis of change, a driving force would be competition. Force field analysis includes:

- Driving forces: These are forces responsible for instigating and promoting change, such as leaders, incentives, and competition.
- Restraining forces: These are forces that resist change, such as poor attitudes, hostility, inadequate equipment, or insufficient funds.

Force field analysis is used when considering changes and begins by listing a proposed change and creating two subgroups below: driving and restraining forces. In order to bring about change, a plan must be developed to diminish or eliminate the restraining forces.

105. A: A cost-benefit analysis uses average cost of a problem (such as wound infections) and the average cost of intervention to demonstrate savings. For example, if a surgical unit averaged 10 surgical site infections annually at an additional average cost of $27,000 each, the total annual cost would be $270,000. If the total cost for interventions, (new staff person, benefits, education, and software) totals $92,000, and the goal is to reduce infections by 50% (0.5 × $270,000 for a total projected savings of $135,000), cost benefit is demonstrated by subtracting the proposed savings from the intervention costs ($135,000 – $92,000) for a savings of $43,000 annually.

106. C: Referring the single mother to a social worker is the most appropriate, as social workers have the expertise required to assist a patient to apply for social services, including programs such as Temporary Assistance for Needy Families (TANF) and food stamps. The social worker may be able to help the patient avoid homelessness by assisting her to apply for subsidized or low-cost housing. While the patient may benefit from a referral to a mental health clinic, this will not solve the immediate underlying problem of food and shelter.

107. D: In providing care to a client, the best approach to encourage client engagement is to ask the client about his or her preferences for treatment. The client should take an active part in discussions about the best methods to deal with the client's diagnosis or situation. Client input into the treatment plan is an essential factor in engagement because the client is more likely to adhere to treatment if he or she has had a voice in the decision making.

108. A: During a partial hospitalization, a patient spends at least four hours daily in a structured setting receiving psychotherapy and milieu therapy. Ambulatory care is outpatient treatment for patients that do not need a structured setting.

109. A: If a 46-year-old male client with type 2 diabetes had been noncompliant with treatment and was switched from oral medications to insulin 3 months earlier but now claims to be compliant with diet and medications, the finding of most concern is an A1c of 8.5 because this indicates that the client's diabetes is uncontrolled. The FBS is also elevated, but not remarkedly so. The A1c reflects what has been happening over a 3-month period and not just the day of the test. The client's BMI is only slightly elevated (normal 18.5 to 24.9), and the BP is within normal values.

110. B: Sometimes patients oppose treatment due to inadequate understanding of clinical information and treatment options. Before proceeding with other actions, the case manager should ensure that the patient has a complete understanding. Discussions and decisions are carefully documented in the chart.

111. A: The theory of reasoned action is based on the idea that the actions people take voluntarily can be predicted according to their personal attitude toward the action and their perception of how others will view their doing the action. The three basic concepts of the theory include:

- Attitudes: Personal attitudes about an action
- Subjective norms: Attitudes of others in the client's social realm
- Behavioral intention: The intention to take action is based on weighing attitudes and subjective norms

112. C: The basic life support ambulance is the appropriate form of transportation for a psychiatric or suicidal patient or those whose care must be monitored, because attendants are available. Private automobiles, usually belonging to family or friends, may be used for stable patients if the patient can be transported and handled safely and if necessary, equipment (such as portable oxygen) is available. Wheelchair vans may be appropriate for people, such as quadriplegics, who are normally confined to wheelchairs. Advanced life support ambulances are used for those with unstable conditions and all those with open intravenous lines or those requiring medications during transportation.

113. B: If a 68-year-old client with renal failure and low income states that her daughter has died of a narcotic overdose, and the client must assume care of three grandchildren but has no idea how to manage this, the most appropriate referral is to a social worker. The social worker will be able to help the client determine whether she is eligible for welfare assistance or other benefits to help pay for the care of the grandchildren and to help the client apply for benefits.

114. B: A PPO is an insurance model that offers patients a preferred panel of physicians. A patient may choose to utilize an "outside" physician, but this would result in lower reimbursement and a greater cost to the patient member. HMOs use physicians as gatekeepers.

115. A: A comprehensive plan for reintegration is critical to success when reintegrating a brain-injured patient back into the community. Issues should include housing, financial support, job training, family support, medical support, assistive devices, environmental modifications, safety, and follow-up. Goals must be realistic with timeframes and based on the patient's activities and skill set before injury/illness as well as any current limitations. Support is especially important during the transition phase while the patient learns to function in a more independent environment. The case manager must be aware of all available services and make necessary referrals.

116. B: Transitions of care generally require handoff/handover of a patient from one level of care to another with responsibility for the patient's care transitioning from one person/place to another. This may occur within one facility when a patient moves from one unit to another or between two facilities. In some cases, multiple handoffs/handovers may occur. Transitions of care may also involve a change in the plan of care or a change in the payor/health plan.

117. B: In a managed healthcare plan, a gag clause prevents healthcare providers from discussing with the patient treatment options that are not covered by that particular managed care plan.

118. A: Case managers often create dashboards to assist in meeting case management goals, patient needs, and the needs of other case management clients. By using dashboard reports, one can determine whether or not a case management department is progressing its efforts to improve. It is similar to a report card.

119. A: If a client who fell and fractured a hip asks if he should limit ambulation to reduce the risk of further falls, the best approach is to discuss the risks of ambulation versus the benefits. It's impossible to eliminate all risks, but the case manager can stress safety measures to reduce the risk and point out that limiting ambulation may lead to increased weakness, which can also increase the risk of fall, whereas ambulation may increase strength and stability.

120. D: While all of these are important, the primary reason for stratifying risk is to provide preventive intervention before problems arise. During risk stratification, clients who are at high risk of incurring rehospitalizations or increased medical costs are identified and intervention plans made to ensure that the client has adequate follow up and treatment in order to reduce utilization of health care services. Clients are placed into high-risk, moderate-risk, or low-risk categories.

121. B: The goals of the ADA include full participation, equal opportunity, independent living, and economic self-sufficiency. Individuals must submit to a case-by-case assessment in order to prove that their impairment is covered under ADA. Proof of a medical diagnosis is no longer sufficient.

122. B: When patients have two or more health plans, the case manager should initially determine which plan provides primary coverage and which provides secondary coverage and so on. Rules vary widely regarding the order of payment, so the case manager may need to contact the health plans and determine the order of insurance responsibility on an individual basis. Double coverage is usually precluded, and the patient is often not able to choose. Medicare is primary over supplementary insurances, and private insurances are primary over Medicaid.

123. A: Appeals for denial of urgent care must be decided by the insurance company within 72 hours. Insurance companies have 30 days to review and make a decision about nonurgent care that a patient has not yet received but 60 days for care that the patient has already received. A patient can appeal directly to their insurance companies if care is denied or ruled medically unnecessary and if the insurance company claims the patient is not eligible, treatment is experimental, or the patient is filing claims for a preexisting condition that is not covered.

124. A: Clinical pathways help standardize care for a particular diagnosis. The pathways are multidisciplinary in nature and often significantly improve outcomes. Pathways include a timeline for providing interventions, whereas guidelines typically do not follow strict timelines.

125. C: Indemnity insurance pays in the form of predetermined payments for loss or damages rather than for healthcare service. Liability insurance pays damages for bodily injury or loss of property, such as injury resulting from unsafe conditions. No-fault auto insurance pays for injury/damages resulting from driving a car, with coverage varying according to state regulations. Accident and health insurance pays for healthcare costs and may or may not include disability payments, depending on the type of policy.

126. C: The strengths-based model of case management focuses on the needs of patients by empowering the patient and their support system with the information and resources they need to take control of their own care. The case manager is responsible for identifying specific needs and coordinating care with various providers while also directing the patient to community resources. By focusing on the strengths of the patient, the case manager empowers the patient to take control of their own care with access to the required support systems.

127. D: If the organization is using the John Hopkins ACG® (Adjusted Clinical Group) system, the case manager expects that it will help to predict clients' future health needs. This system considers all of the client's morbidity and healthcare history and experiences rather than the practice pattern of the clinician when assessing risk. The ACG system helps to better identify those clients who are at risk for further health problems and may benefit from case management and interventions.

128. A: A Current Procedural Terminology (CPT) code is a numeric code that describes a diagnostic, medical, or surgical service. CPT codes describe uniform information about medical services and procedures for the benefit of physicians, coders, and payers. ICD-10 codes are alphanumeric designations that represent diseases or conditions.

129. D: A Medicare Advantage Plan (MAP) is approved by Medicare but administered by private insurance companies. These plans must follow the rules established by Medicare. Medicare pays a fixed amount per month to the insurance company for beneficiaries who are enrolled. A MAP is a form of managed care, so while all of the services provided under Medicare Parts A and B are covered, the MAP may offer additional services, such as dental and vision care, but offers less flexibility since healthcare providers must be chosen from a network, and preapproval is required for treatment.

130. A: As a case manager in a nurse-family partnership, an appropriate intervention includes providing information about smoking cessation and abstinence from drugs. This program targets low-income first-time parents in order to prevent pregnancy complications through changing maternal behaviors (smoking, drug and alcohol use), improving the health and development of the child by helping parents develop parenting skills, and helping the parents to develop self-sufficiency (family planning, education, work).

131. D: This is an example of patient self-determination. In this process, the patient makes treatment decisions such as establishing advance directives, appointing a healthcare proxy, determining whether to withdraw nutrition, or electing not to be resuscitated.

132. C: When a billing code makes a patient seems more severely ill than he really is, upcoding has occurred. Upcoding is sometimes done intentionally to increase reimbursement, but it can also be done accidentally by an inexperienced coder. Consistently upcoding constitutes fraud.

133. A: An FROI is written by the employer to report a work-related injury to begin the process of filing a workers' compensation claim. Employers are not trained to do functional capacity exams or to provide an impairment rating. Impairment ratings are based on the findings of a physician.

134. D: Residential care facilities (also called assisted living facilities) are similar to apartment buildings with private suites. Some of the characteristics include wheelchair accessibility, higher toilets, and communications devices. Adult day care offers care outside the home as a temporary alternative for caregivers. Green houses are group homes focusing on quality of life. Skilled nursing facilities provide medical care.

135. D: Rewards for more expensive plans. Accountable care organizations, quality reporting, and chronic disease management are cornerstones of the PPACA. Part of the PPACA includes a "Cadillac tax" (beginning 2018) for expensive health care plans. This is meant to decrease the cost of healthcare by reducing availability of these types of plans. Of note, most of these "Cadillac" plans are paid for by employers and the patients never deal with the costs of the healthcare plan. Therefore, when these plans are less available patients will be more acutely aware of the cost of healthcare.

136. B: A right of subrogation clause allows insurance plans to pay for initial treatment until payor responsibility is ascertained. Coordination of benefits lets payors decrease payments by the amount of coverage provided by another medical insurance policy. An indemnity is a form of commercial medical insurance whereby the patient pays a deductible and a percentage of costs.

137. C: The Tuberculosis Medicaid program provided by the DSS is intended to provide coverage for evaluation and treatment of TB, including medications and directly observed therapy (DOT) for those patients who are uninsured or underinsured and do not qualify for regular Medicaid. To qualify, patients must be citizens or legal residents and must have resided in the United States for at least five years. Patients who have insurance but no coverage for DOT may be covered under this program for daily DOT.

138. C: The first step in the interview process should be to establish rapport with the client. In emergency situations, this may not be possible, but in most situations taking 1–2 minutes to chat with the client, ensure that the client is comfortable, and offer water can help the client relax and reduce his or her stress. If a client feels comfortable, he or she will be more amenable to questioning and sharing personal information.

139. A: Medical home models encourage a proactive and planned approach to health care. The primary care physician is at the center of the model along with involvement of the nonphysician staff.

140. A: The purpose of stop-loss insurance, a form of reinsurance, is to protect an insurance company against excessive payments. Thus, the primary insurance may cover the first $150,000 of medical bills, and then the stop-loss insurance pays a percentage (usually around 80 percent) of bills over that amount, with the primary insurance paying the remainder (usually around 20 percent). Stop-loss is especially valuable for smaller self-funded insurance plans.

141. C: If the case manager reviews clients' records and notes that there are numerous examples of deviations from evidence-based guidelines and tries to assess the reason, this is an example of risk management. Deviating from evidence-based guidelines can increase the risks of complications and can result in substandard care. Identifying a pattern of such deviations suggests that staff are not adequately trained or are negligent, there are systemic problems that prevent compliance, or staff are uninformed about the importance of consistently following the guidelines.

142. D: If an 18-year-old homeschooled client with cystic fibrosis is at her first semester away from home in college, but has been hospitalized for respiratory infections twice, gained 5 pounds, and needed a change in medications, the case manager recognizes the client most needs education from the pulmonologist. The client must understand the risk from close associations with others and preventive measures to take to reduce the risk of infection. The client has likely been on many medications throughout her life, so a change is common. A five-pound weight gain is also common for those at college for the first time.

143. C: Interdisciplinary palliative care teams ensure that providers from multiple specialties (e.g., physician, social worker, nurse, chaplain) can collaborate with the patient and family to craft a care plan that meets the needs and goals of the patient. Care is directed primarily by the patient. Ideally, the team provides information and elicits patient values, preferences, and goals as they pertain to end-of-life care. Once this is completed, specific challenges can be identified and possible solutions planned. Interventions are then provided to the patient and family in accordance with the formulated plan. Reassessments and changes in the care plan are made as illness progresses or preferences or goals change.

144. B: Patients under subacute care don't need diagnostic work-ups. Subacute care includes all levels of care not requiring acute hospitalization. The patients are medically stable and have a constant treatment plan.

145. D: Preparation. Transtheoretical stages:

- Precontemplation: Client informed about consequences of problem behavior and has no intention of changing behavior in the next 6 months.
- Contemplation: Client aware of costs and benefits of changing behavior and intends to change in the next 6 months but is procrastinating.
- Preparation: Client has a plan to instigate change in the near future (≤1 month) and is ready for action plans.
- Action: Client modifies behavior. Change occurs only if behavior meets a set criterion (such as complete abstinence from drinking).
- Maintenance: Client works to maintain changes and gains confidence that he/she will not relapse.

146. C: The legal document that designates someone to make decisions regarding medical and end-of-life care if a patient is mentally incompetent is a Durable Power of Attorney for Health Care. This is one type of advance directive, which can also include a living will, a medical power of attorney, and other specific requests of the patient regarding his or her health care. A do-not-resuscitate order is a physician-generated document that is completed when a patient does not want resuscitative treatment in an end-of-life situation. A general power of attorney allows a designated person to make decisions for a person over broader areas, including financial concerns.

147. C: The scenario describes intermediate care. Under assisted living or custodial care, the client is stable, takes a consistent regimen of oral medications, and does not need suctioning. Skilled nursing is for complex, but generally stable, patients who may need central line care, IV push medications, variable adjustments in dosages of medicines, and assessment of laboratory values.

148. A: While criteria may vary for admission to case management, a primary indication of need is a client with 6 or more visits to an emergency department in the past 12 months, especially if any visits occurred in the previous 6 months. Repeated ED visits indicate that the client's medical condition is not under good control or is not being managed appropriately by the client. Other indications may include two or more admissions to a hospital in the past year with one in the last 6 months, and a client who is under the care of 3 or more specialists and experiences polypharmacy.

149. B: Under Medicare, the eligibility for home health care includes being "homebound," but this does not literally mean the patient is never able to leave home. The patient may leave the home with assistance (wheelchair, walker, special transportation) for short periods for medical (doctor's office visit, therapy) or nonmedical purposes (such as attending church). Patients are considered homebound if a physician recommends the patient not leave the home because of a condition (such as TB) or if leaving the home requires difficult effort.

150. C: Conformance costs include those related to preventing errors, such as monitoring and evaluation. Nonconformance costs are those related to errors, failures, and defects. These may include adverse events (such as infections), poor access due to staff shortages or cancellations, lost time, duplications of service, and malpractice. Error-free costs are all those costs in terms of processes, services, equipment, time, materials, and staffing that are necessary to providing a product or process that is without error from the onset. Indirect costs are shared costs, such as infrastructure costs and the cost of custodial services.

151. C: If an 87-year-old client with leukemia and renal failure has developed a severe respiratory infection but has refused mechanical ventilation, the case manager should remain supportive and ensure that the client receive comfort care. Because the client already has two life-threatening conditions, the client's quality of life and chances of recovery should be considered. As long as the client is able to make an informed consent, the client has the legal right to refuse any treatment.

152. B: If a 76-year-old stroke client with left-sided weakness is being discharged from a rehabilitation center and insists on returning home under the care of her daughter, who has had no experience in caregiving, the most helpful referral is likely an occupational therapist. The OT can observe the client and caregiver doing tasks and assess needs and may help the client develop compensatory skills and suggest modifications to the home environment and assistive devices. The OT can educate the daughter about methods of caring for the client.

153. A: Critical pathways are grids depicting the key events expected to occur on each day of a patient's hospitalization. They are also known as critical paths.

154. D: Spend down is the process by which people spend down assets on medical bills to qualify for Medicaid. Medicaid is administered by states, so regulations vary, but in order to qualify, people must be low income. However, if they have inadequate or no insurance, they can deduct the costs (paid or unpaid bills) they have incurred for medical services from their excess income in order to qualify. Once the spend down reaches the income requirement, Medicaid will pay the remaining medical bills.

155. B: The case manager should suspect that the client most at risk for dual diagnosis is a client with bipolar disease, other mental health disease (such as schizophrenia), or PTSD. These clients often go without diagnosis or treatment for prolonged periods and tend to rely on drugs and alcohol as a means to self-medicate. Therefore, in addition to treatment for their mental health issues, the clients are likely in need of specialized drug/alcohol rehabilitation.

156. B: When educating a client, a technique that most optimizes engagement is having the client do teach-back. Engagement refers to the client's involvement in provision of self-care to improve outcomes. With teach-back, the CMM provides education and demonstration and then observes the client explaining the procedure while carrying out the steps to the procedure. The role of the case manager is to provide feedback and encouragement to the client and help to build the client's self-confidence. Clients are more likely to feel confident about the steps to a procedure if they have taught it to someone else.

157. C: Timelines for multidisciplinary action plans vary depending on the patient's clinical needs. It could be hours, days, weeks, or months. A CareMap for a 24-week- gestation infant could be several months. Variance time frames must also be determined, including determining how much leeway should be allowed for achieving the expected outcomes.

158. D: If there is a possible conflict of interest in working with a patient, report it to the supervisor so that another case manager can take the assignment. A case manager should never place himself or herself in personal danger in order to provide services. Again, report dangerous conditions to the supervisor.

159. A: Characteristics of a skilled nursing facility (SNF) include physicians are required to visit frequently, but not daily, and a physician extender (nurse practitioner, physician's assistant) may visit instead of the physician. Care is primarily driven by nursing rather than physicians, and lab, pharmacy, and radiology services must be available but are not required to be onsite. Respiratory therapy must be available for clients, but a therapist does not have to be available onsite around the clock.

160. C: The case closure domain focuses on ending the case manager-client relationship and on notification of service termination to stakeholders. Obtaining client consent for services refers to the case finding and intake domain. Utilization review refers to the utilization management domain. The ability of a caregiver to perform necessary services refers to the psychosocial domain.

161. C: Adult Children of Alcoholics (ACOA) is specifically intended for adults who grew up in a home with an alcoholic. Al-Anon is more encompassing and includes all family members of a person with alcoholism. Alateen is a program for adolescents with an alcoholic parent. These are twelve-step programs associated with Alcoholics Anonymous. Children Are People is a program for school-aged children who have a family member who is alcoholic. This program targets at-risk children and provides various services, including tutoring, mentoring, and counseling.

162. D: Under the 60 percent rule, 13 medical conditions qualify. Those that require additional clinical criteria beyond diagnosis include severe osteoarthritis, systemic vasculitides, other arthritis conditions (active polyarticular, psoriatic, and seronegative arthropathia) and complex knee and/or hip joint replacement. The other conditions (based on diagnosis) include stroke, spinal cord injury, hip fracture, brain injury, congenital deformity, amputation, major multiple traumas, burns, and neurological disorders (multiple sclerosis, motor neuron disease, muscular dystrophy, polyneuropathy, and Parkinson's disease).

163. C: While all of these are important, preventing complications after a spinal cord injury is critical because development of complications may severely limit independence and impair psychological well-being and may be life threatening. Common complications include pressure sores, urinary tract infections, deep vein thrombosis, pulmonary emboli, pneumonia, and autonomic dysreflexia. Pressure sores can lead to severe systemic infection. Heterotropic ossification, especially of the hips, can be overlooked until it is advanced but can result in impaired ROM and mobility.

164. C: Activities of home management that a person performs on a regular basis such as housework and meal preparation are instrumental activities of daily living. Activities of daily living are activities that are a part of normal daily living such as eating, bathing, and toileting. Cognitive activities stimulate brain function. On the other hand, executive functions are cognitive abilities that allow a person to prioritize and plan.

165. A: If a client with long-term diabetes mellitus type 1 and an insulin pump has been running high FBSs and made 4 recent trips to the emergency room despite insisting that he is following the diet and proper procedures for the pump and has been using the same abdominal site, the case manager should advise the client to rotate needle insertion sites. Scar tissue can build up at the site of injection if the same site is used repeatedly, and this can affect the absorption of the insulin.

166. D: Objectivity: According to the Code of Professional Conduct for Case Managers principles, case managers should:

- Place public interest above their own.
- Respect the rights and dignity of clients.
- Maintain objectivity.
- Act with integrity and fidelity.
- Maintain competency.
- Honor the profession and CCM designation.
- Obey all laws and regulations.
- Help review and revise the code.

167. D: Poverty has the greatest impact on the incidence of depression, with those in poverty having a rate of about 31% compared to about 16% for those not in poverty. The rate of hypertension is slightly higher among those living in poverty, but rates of cancer and high cholesterol are actually slightly higher in populations that do not live in poverty. If caring for clients in poverty, the case manager should screen the individuals for depression because this may affect their ability and motivation to comply with treatment.

168. A: Credentialing protects the client by ensuring that individuals hired to practice case management are capable of providing quality service. It involves reviewing competencies, licensure, history of malpractice, and other parameters. Certification is a credential awarded by a certifying agency to a person who meets certification criteria by passing an examination. Accreditation is granted by a nationally recognized agency to a healthcare organization that meets required standards. Licensure affirms that a person has the basic knowledge and skills to practice a profession.

169. C: The first step in developing a healthcare management program is to define the population to be served. This usually derives from data regarding those with similar diagnoses, risks for complications, frequent need for clinical services, and/or high-cost interventions. The program is then developed with the goal, such as reducing costs or reducing complications, in mind. Barriers should be identified and strategies, including resources and different options, developed to implement the plan as well as methods for measuring outcomes.

170. D: One of the components of case management is client identification and outreach. Clients who need case management services must be identified. Entry into a case management program involves an interview process, a referral, or networking systems. A case manager may also promote eligibility for certain individuals.

171. C: There are six domains for case management practice. These include psychosocial concepts and support systems; care delivery and reimbursement methods; quality and outcomes evaluation and measurement; rehabilitation concepts and strategies; ethical, legal and practice standards; and professional development and advancement. Risk management is a subdomain of quality and outcomes evaluation and measurement.

172. B: Medicare Select requires use of specific providers, so it is a form of managed care. Provider lists can include hospitals as well as physicians. Patients who receive care outside of this network generally do not receive full benefits or may even be denied benefits, although some forms of emergency care may be covered. Medicare Select offers the same 12 basic programs as Medigap insurance, but premiums are usually lower because patients have less flexibility in accessing health care.

173. C: A functional capacity evaluation includes grading strength activities, position tolerance activities, and mobility activities. It also includes a review of the medical record and evaluation of the musculoskeletal system. Literacy screening is not a component of the functional capacity evaluation.

174. A: Force field analysis is a decision-making technique that comprises both consideration of restraining forces, which negatively impact a program, and driving forces, which positively impact the program. Restraining forces can include satisfaction with the status quo (or fear of change), lack of support from administration, lack of adequate resources, inadequate numbers of staff, lack of time, lack of knowledge, and fear of statistics. Driving forces can include the need or desire to predict needed skill sets, track present and future costs, improve outcomes, and remain current.

175. A: The question defines a per-diem reimbursement in which a predetermined fixed rate is established for each day of hospitalization and then reimbursed to the patient according to length of hospital stay. A cost-based reimbursement refers to actual costs of a patient's care. In fee for service, the provider bills the insurance company and the company pays for services. Capitation is a fixed monthly payment paid to a provider in advance of services.

176. B: The only goal-oriented activity listed here is to start IV antibiotics within two hours of admission if not already started in the ED. Checking oxygen saturations and baseline mental status are assessments. Obtaining a pulmonary consult and determining educational needs are under the category of consults and multidisciplinary education. Administration of antipyretics and pain meds are therapy.

177. D: If a 72-year-old client with COPD was discharged from an acute hospital after a bout of pneumonia and has orders for low-dose oxygen 24 hours a day, but when the case manager telephones, the client seems unclear about when or how to use the oxygen or equipment, the most appropriate referral is to a home health agency. The home health nurse can evaluate the client's condition and provide education about the use of oxygen and the equipment.

178. A: If a confused elderly client shows extensive bruising and flinches and appears fearful when approached by family members and the case manager suspects elder abuse, the case manager should report possible abuse to adult protective services for evaluation. Unless the abuse is obvious and severe (e.g., broken bones, etc.) and the client may be at risk of immediate further injury, the police are not usually notified of suspected abuse by those reporting it.

179. B: Advocacy is working for the best interests of the patient despite conflicting personal values and assisting patients to have access to appropriate resources. Moral agency is the ability to recognize needs and a willingness take action to influence the wholesome outcome of a conflict or decision. Agency is a general willingness to act arising from openness and the recognition of involved issues. Collaboration is working together to achieve better results.

180. C: If a case manager suggests a change in procedure and other staff members fail to discuss the proposed change or take any actions regarding it, this indicates passive rejection. Active rejection occurs when a change is purposefully rejected, such as by a vote after discussion. In order to avoid passive rejection, it may be important to suggest a change in a formal way, such as placing it on a meeting agenda for discussion and going to the meeting prepared with data to support the change.

CCM Practice Test #2

1. In assisted living facilities, staffing must include:

a. 24-hour staffing (skilled or unskilled).
b. 24-hour skilled nursing.
c. 12-hour skilled nursing and 12-hour unskilled.
d. 12-hour staffing (skilled or unskilled).

2. A situation that may be perceived as a conflict of interest is if the case manager:

a. Provides clients with a list of local physical therapists, which includes the physical therapy practice of the case manager's brother-in-law
b. Refers clients to a physical therapy practice run by the case manager's brother-in-law
c. Picks up the case of a client who attends physical therapy at the case manager's brother-in-law's practice
d. Lives in the same neighborhood as the client but has seen the client only in passing

3. The most useful way in which to divide groups of clients is by:

a. Risk stratification.
b. Projected costs.
c. Gender.
d. Ethnicity/Cultural background.

4. If a $100,000 investment in hiring a case manager results in savings of $120,000, then $20,000 represents the:

a. Capital gains.
b. Profit.
c. Return on investment.
d. Avoidable costs.

5. The average length of stay in an acute care hospital for a client 65 to 84 years of age with septicemia is approximately:

a. 5 to 7 days.
b. 8 to 10 days.
c. 11 to 14 days.
d. 15 to 20 days.

6. If the client chooses to forego transfer to an inpatient rehabilitation center and have home health care instead against the advice of the physician and the case manager, and the case manager alters the plan of care to correspond with the client's wishes, the case manager is exhibiting the ethical principle of:

a. Beneficence.
b. Autonomy.
c. Nonmaleficence.
d. Justice.

7. In dealing with conflict, a staff person who follows the guidelines of the case manager he or she disagrees with is exhibiting:

a. Accommodation.
b. Compromise.
c. Avoidance.
d. Collaboration.

8. If a case manager works with a second case manager and has observed the second case manager falsifying records of contacts that the second case manager did not actually make, the correct action is to:

a. Immediately report the situation to the supervisor/employer.
b. Confront the second case manager about the practice.
c. Offer to help the second case manager with the contacts.
d. Avoid working with the second case manager.

9. If a client was seriously injured at work but feels that the employer was negligent and plans to sue, the client should:

a. Apply for workers' compensation and then file suit.
b. File suit and then apply for workers' compensation.
c. Wait before making any type of decision.
d. File suit and avoid applying for workers' compensation.

10. When completing a cost-benefit analysis, an example of a "soft" cost savings is:

a. Decreased length of hospitalization stay.
b. Prevention of complications.
c. Client's change to a provider in the network.
d. Transfer from lower level of care.

11. Prior to the initial interview with a client, the case manager should:

a. Review the client's medical records.
b. Interview the client's nursing staff.
c. Review the client's insurance plan.
d. Assess the client's ability to pay any necessary costs.

12. If a client in an acute care hospital is stable but will require 7 further days of IV antibiotics during recovery from surgery and a severe post-operative infection, the most appropriate level of care is:

a. Long-term acute care facility.
b. Skilled nursing facility.
c. Subacute care facility.
d. Acute care hospital.

13. Under the hospice benefit for end-of-life care, *home* is defined as:

a. The client's primary residence.
b. The client's primary residence or a skilled nursing facility.
c. Any place the client is residing.
d. The client's primary residence or any licensed health care facility.

14. The passive acquisition of cases refers to:

a. Routine acquisition of all of one category of client.
b. Acquisition based on client request.
c. Acquisition based on direct observation of need.
d. Acquisition by referral from health care providers.

15. A person who was injured on the job and unable to work for 3 months would receive Workers' Compensation benefits at the level of:

a. Permanent total disability (PTD).
b. Temporary partial disability (TPD).
c. Permanent partial impairment (PPI).
d. Temporary total disability (TTD).

16. Under the Health Insurance Portability and Accountability Act (HIPAA) regulations, clients who request copies of laboratory results must receive them within:

a. 24 hours.
b. 48 hours.
c. 14 days.
d. 30 days.

17. A discharge planning evaluation must include an evaluation of the:

a. Client's need for post-hospitalization services.
b. Projected costs of post-hospitalization services.
c. Community agencies available.
d. Client's cognitive abilities.

18. The CMS Clinical Quality Measures, in their Adult Recommended Core Measures, recommend that screening for depression (NQF 0418) begin at age:

a. 12 years.
b. 14 years.
c. 18 years.
d. 21 years.

19. If a client on Medicare requires durable medical equipment, the costs should be covered by:

a. Medicare A.
b. Medicare B.
c. Medicare C.
d. Medicare D.

20. An example of an emergent group is:

a. Legislative body.
b. Research team.
c. Social agency.
d. Group of friends.

21. Focused utilization management programs that target only specific client populations often result in:

a. Cost savings and improved care.
b. Care deficiencies.
c. Skewed data and inaccurate interpretation of data.
d. Time and cost savings.

22. The National Quality Forum's CMS readmission measures cover all of the following EXCEPT:

a. Pulmonary embolism.
b. Heart attack and heart failure.
c. Pneumonia.
d. COPD and knee/hip replacement.

23. An indemnity insurance plan is usually an example of:

a. HMO.
b. Fee-for-service.
c. PPO.
d. POS.

24. If a client was injured at work and is undergoing rehabilitation for physical strengthening 2 days a week in preparation for returning to work, this is referred to as:

a. Work hardening.
b. Work conditioning.
c. Work preparation.
d. Work adjustment.

25. When the client of a mental health case manager refuses case management after being discharged from a mental institution, the case manager should:

a. Assess the need for court-ordered case management.
b. Try to convince the client to have case management.
c. Allow the client to refuse services.
d. Refer the client to the public health department.

26. A swing bed agreement with CMS allows a hospital to:

a. Move a client from one room to another.
b. Place clients in Stryker frames to facilitate change in position.
c. Use the same bed for acute or skilled nursing facility care.
d. Have some beds without any type of side rails.

27. When doing case management evaluation using the cost-effectiveness analysis method, *sensitivity analysis* refers to:

a. Determining who pays and who benefits.
b. Timing of accrual of costs and benefits.
c. Specifying types of costs.
d. Testing assumptions and validating conclusions.

28. If a client's insurance is an exclusive provider organization (EPO) and the client chooses to see a physician outside of the network and receives a bill for $500, the client must pay:

a. 20%.
b. 50%.
c. 80%.
d. 100%.

29. For payer-based case management services, contact with the client is usually via:

a. Face-to-face contact
b. Telephone
c. Video
d. Written communication

30. The Digit Repetition Test is primarily used to diagnose:

a. Early dementia.
b. Depression.
c. Delirium.
d. Attention deficits.

31. A terminally ill client who believes that prayer will heal her probably:

a. Is in a state of denial.
b. Is delusional.
c. Depends on faith for comfort.
d. Needs education about her disease.

32. When a client has signed a release of information form so the case manager can provide information to a therapist, the case manager should:

a. Release all available information.
b. Ask the client, item by item, what should be released.
c. Release the minimum information necessary to meet the request.
d. Edit the information released to the therapist.

33. In order for an organization to receive health plan accreditation from the National Committee for Quality Assurance (NCQA), the organization must report and meet measures of performance that are divided into 6 standards of focus. These standards include all of the following EXCEPT:

a. Outcome evaluation.
b. Member experience.
c. Population health management.
d. Network management.

34. A client who is a devoutly religious Catholic and believes her health problems are punishment for sins may benefit most from:

a. Self-help groups.
b. Pastoral counseling.
c. Self-help literature.
d. Psychotherapy.

35. The score for the REALM (Rapid Estimate of Adult Literacy in Medicine) test is based on the:

a. Number of words the client can define.
b. Number of questions the client can answer correctly.
c. Number of words the client can pronounce.
d. Number of words the client can spell.

36. The case manager expects that a client with a Karnofsky Performance Status Scale score of 30 will require:

a. No special intervention.
b. Occasional assistance with personal care.
c. Institutional or hospital care.
d. Frequent assistance with personal care.

37. Palliative care is intended for those who:

a. Have specific diagnoses, such as cancer or heart disease.
b. No longer have curative treatments.
c. Need to improve the quality of life by managing symptoms.
d. Need comfort care during the last 6 months of life.

38. The case manager who wants to justify further intervention for a rehabilitation client who has not met performance goals should begin with:

a. The data on admission to the program.
b. Current data related to ability to perform.
c. An explanation of performance goals.
d. An overview of benefits allowed for the client in their insurance plan.

39. When considering whether the Americans with Disabilities Act will provide protections for a client, the case manager recognizes that a condition that may be considered a disability is:

a. Pyromania.
b. Compulsive gambling.
c. Alcoholism.
d. Kleptomania.

40. In a payer-based case management model, the case manager is generally an employee of the:

a. Physician.
b. Agency providing care.
c. Client.
d. Insurance company.

41. The primary purpose of admission certification is to determine:

a. The correct diagnostic-related group (DRG) for the client.
b. The client's maximal insurance benefit.
c. The client's projected cost for hospitalization.
d. The medical necessity of admission.

42. The FOCUS (find, organize, clarify, uncover, start) performance improvement model to facilitate change is primarily used to:

a. Develop solutions.
b. Evaluate outcomes.
c. Identify problems.
d. Implement programs.

43. The most common reasons for screening clients to determine need for case management are:

a. Diagnosis, high rates of resource utilization, and high costs of care.
b. Diagnosis, age, and high rates of resource utilization.
c. Diagnosis, age, and high costs of care.
d. Diagnosis, high rates of resource utilization, and projected length of stay.

44. When preparing a quality improvement report, the case manager should begin with:

a. An outline of interventions.
b. The indicator that was measured.
c. The type of measurement used for assessment.
d. The results of the intervention.

45. A physical disability would include:

a. Blindness.
b. Deafness.
c. Osteoarthritis in knees.
d. Balance disorder.

46. In an acute care hospital interdisciplinary team, the individual primarily responsible for assessing the post-discharge needs of the client is the:

a. Physician.
b. Case manager.
c. Social worker.
d. Occupational therapist.

47. To prevent back injury when standing on the floor and lifting heavy items, the items should be:

a. 30 to 40 inches above the floor.
b. At waist level.
c. At knee level.
d. 20 to 30 inches above the floor.

48. The purpose of a concurrent review of a hospitalized client is to assess:

a. The client's medical necessity for admission.
b. The need for prescribed treatments.
c. The need for continued hospitalization.
d. The client's need for discharge planning.

49. In Roberts' Seven-Stage Crisis Intervention Model, the first stage includes:

a. Assessing lethality.
b. Establishing rapport.
c. Identifying major problems/precipitants.
d. Exploring alternatives.

50. The health maintenance organization (HMO) model that allows individual or groups of physicians to contract with an HMO to provide services while also seeing non-HMO clients is:

a. Staff model.
b. Independent practice association (IPA).
c. Group practice.
d. Direct contract.

51. The best response to a client who is progressing well after a stroke but remains extremely fearful and anxious about discharge is to:

a. Explore the client's concerns with the client.
b. Reassure the client that everything will be all right.
c. Refer the client to a psychologist.
d. Delay discharge until the client feels ready.

52. RotaCare clinics provide free medical care to:

a. Clients who are homeless only.
b. Clients who are uninsured, underinsured, and/or homeless.
c. Diabetic clients only.
d. Infants and children only.

53. The primary purpose of a benchmark study is to identify:

a. Best practices.
b. Gaps in performance.
c. Cost-saving measures.
d. Areas for further research.

54. An elderly low-income home care client who is losing weight because she doesn't like to cook and lives on junk food may benefit most from:

a. Meal delivery services.
b. Admission to an assisted living facility.
c. Referral to a nutritionist.
d. Homemaker services.

55. Insurance companies hire case managers primarily to:

a. Provide the best care possible.
b. Reduce costs of care.
c. Educate the client.
d. Investigate claims.

56. Statements that outline the level of performance expected of a professional, such as a case manager, are included in:

a. Case management plans.
b. Standards of care.
c. Evidence-based practice guidelines.
d. Standards of practice.

57. The model of acute care case management that follows the client's progress through acute hospitalization to ensure effective, safe, and cost-effective transition from acute care to post-acute care is:

a. Integrated functions.
b. Disease management.
c. Clinical resources.
d. Outcomes management.

58. A TRICARE beneficiary is eligible for TRICARE for Life if the person has:

a. Medicare A.
b. Medicare B.
c. Medicare A and B.
d. no Medicare.

59. A client who would have been eligible for Medicaid in January but does not apply until June first is entitled to coverage that starts:

a. January 1.
b. June 1.
c. March 1.
d. May 1.

60. The TRICARE program that utilizes a preferred provider organization (PPO) is:

a. TRICARE Standard.
b. TRICARE Extra.
c. TRICARE Prime.
d. TRICARE Reserve Select.

61. An individual purchasing an insurance plan through an exchange should expect that a silver tier plan will pay:

a. 90% of medical expenses.
b. 80% of medical expenses.
c. 70% of medical expenses.
d. 60% of medical expenses.

62. Under Medicare Part A and/or Part B, the home health services that are covered include:

a. Homemaker service.
b. Round-the-clock care in the home.
c. Meals delivered to the home.
d. Intermittent skilled nursing care.

63. The best placement for a 24-year-old client with schizophrenia being discharged from a psychiatric institution for the first time in 4 years is likely:

a. Skilled nursing facility.
b. Private apartment.
c. Shared apartment.
d. Group home.

64. The billing code that is utilized for services such as ambulance and durable medical equipment is:

a. ICD-10-CM.
b. ICD-10-PCS.
c. CPT-4.
d. HCPCS-Level II.

65. A series of steps in treatment based on client response and developed through scientific and evidence-based research in order to standardize a specific type of care is referred to as a(n):

a. Protocol.
b. Decision tree.
c. Algorithm.
d. Care map.

66. In order to qualify for Medicare based on a 63-year-old spouse's work record, the applicant must be at least:

a. 62 years old.
b. 63 years old.
c. 64 years old.
d. 65 years old.

67. When making decisions about case management based on catastrophic diagnoses, diagnoses would include:

a. Pneumonia.
b. Syncope.
c. Solid-organ transplants.
d. Seizure disorder (new onset).

68. The term that would most apply to a transgender female (biological male) who is sexually attracted to females is:

a. Lesbian.
b. Gay.
c. Bisexual.
d. Heterosexual.

69. A cost-containment strategy in which all clients receiving similar services or treatments from the same provider have the same payment rate is:

a. Episode-of-care payments.
b. Performance-based provider payments (P4P).
c. All-payer rate setting.
d. Global payments.

70. The appropriate referral for a client with swallowing problems following a stroke is:

a. Occupational therapist.
b. Speech therapist.
c. Physical therapist.
d. Nutritionist.

71. A client who remains grief-stricken and depressed 10 months after her husband's death and has been unable to work or care for her family or home would probably benefit most from a:

a. Support group.
b. Psychologist.
c. Bereavement counselor.
d. Psychiatrist.

72. As part of utilization management, the Milliman Care Guideline that is appropriate for clients with complex clinical situations and diagnoses for which a specific guideline does not exist is:

a. General recovery.
b. Chronic care.
c. Inpatient and surgical care.
d. Ambulatory care.

73. The SAFE questions to ask a client suspected of being a victim of abuse include questions about Stress/Safety, Afraid/Abused, Friends/Family, and:

a. Escalation.
b. Emergency plan.
c. Employment.
d. Education.

74. The instrument that is most appropriate to assess general health and disability across all medical disciplines, including mental, neurological, and substance abuse, is:

a. Global Assessment of Functioning (GAF) test.
b. Instrumental Activities of Daily Living (IADL) assessment.
c. The Time and Change test.
d. World Health Organization Disability Assessment Schedule 2 (WHODAS-2).

75. The primary focus of job analysis is on the specific requirements of the:

a. Job.
b. Person.
c. Company.
d. Law/Regulations.

76. The case manager who cannot find food or shelter for a homeless client may receive assistance for the client from the local:

a. Salvation Army.
b. Public Health Department.
c. RotaCare clinic.
d. Medical society.

77. A case manager assigned to a population health program in an African American community with high rates of hypertension and diabetes should initially focus education on:

a. Compliance with treatment.
b. Diet and exercise.
c. BP and glucose monitoring.
d. Drug and alcohol use.

78. The case manager is preparing a client to undergo a functional capacity evaluation required by the client's insurance company following injury and tells the client that the evaluation will not include:

a. Lifting ability.
b. Range of motion.
c. Motivation.
d. Stamina.

79. Disease management programs are usually intended for:

a. Specific population of clients.
b. All clients.
c. Hospitalized clients.
d. Both low- and high-risk clients.

80. Case management information systems (CMISs) generally include:

a. Financial management programs.
b. Standardized plans of care.
c. Computerized physician order entry systems.
d. Pharmacy information systems.

81. If the case manager wants to apply the correct diagnostic code for outpatient services to a billing form, the case manager would utilize:

a. CPT-4.
b. NDC.
c. ICD-10-PCS.
d. ICD-10-CM.

82. The type of managed care plan that allows a client to see physicians and care providers within a network but to seek outside treatment in some circumstances is:

a. Health maintenance organization (HMO).
b. Exclusive provider organization (EPO).
c. Point of service plan (POS).
d. Preferred provider organization (PPO).

83. In negotiating prices with an out-of-network health care provider, the case manager should begin by:

a. Asserting limits to reimbursement.
b. Researching prices.
c. Establishing goals for client care.
d. Appealing to the health care provider's empathy.

84. The focus of case management in a pre-acute environment, such as a physician's office or clinic, is often on:

a. Coordination of providers.
b. Collaboration.
c. Utilization.
d. Prevention.

85. The government entity that requires that personal protective equipment be readily available at the worksite and in appropriate sizes is the:

a. CDC.
b. FDA.
c. OSHA.
d. CMS.

86. When counseling a client, the statement by a case manager that is a misrepresentation of qualifications is:

a. "Your insurance policy excludes payment for this equipment."
b. "You don't need any more physical therapy."
c. "Your income exceeds Medicaid qualifications."
d. "The St. John's wort you are taking can interfere with birth control pills."

87. A rehabilitation center that has received accreditation from the Commission on Accreditation of Rehabilitation Facilities (CARF) indicating the need for improvement in case management must submit a Quality Improvement Plan (QIP) within:

a. 30 days.
b. 60 days.
c. 90 days.
d. 120 days.

88. When a client tells the case manager that her caregiver does not allow her to use the telephone or read her mail, the case manager should suspect that the client is:

a. Confused.
b. Lying.
c. Experiencing psychological abuse.
d. Experiencing neglect.

89. The best solution for working with a client who expresses extreme prejudice toward ethnic minorities and the LGBT population is to:

a. Tell the client his attitude is reprehensible.
b. Refuse to work with the client.
c. Provide professional service and avoid debate.
d. Provide minimal service and avoid interacting with client.

90. The government agency that provides clinical guidelines and recommendations for health care professionals is:

a. CDC.
b. NIH.
c. AHRQ.
d. CMS.

91. Chronic disease in elderly adults is most often associated with:

a. Depression.
b. Dementia.
c. Substance abuse.
d. Partner abuse.

92. When screening the body mass index (BMI) as part of the CMS core measure, what is the acceptable BMI range for a 55-year-old?

a. 18.5-25
b. 18.5-28
c. 20-30
d. 23-30

93. The Blaylock Risk Assessment Screening Score (BRASS) is a tool used to:

a. Identify older adults at risk of prolonged hospitalization.
b. Assess risk of falls in hospitalized clients.
c. Identify clients at risk for hospital-acquired infections.
d. Assess the client's ability to provide self-care on discharge.

94. The FDA will allow emergency use of a drug with filing of an Investigational New Drug (IND) exemption for:

a. One disease/condition only.
b. One client only.
c. No more than 4 clients.
d. A 1-month time period only.

95. Allowing a person to start work 2 hours earlier to accommodate a radiation treatment schedule is an example of:

a. Job modification.
b. Job restructuring.
c. Work hardening.
d. Job analysis.

96. The best tool to combat fear of technology and data is:

a. Education.
b. One-on-one supervision.
c. Clear structure.
d. Consultant.

97. If a person who identifies herself as the client's wife calls and asks for information about a hospitalized client, the case manager should:

a. Provide the information the person requests.
b. Make arrangements to meet with the client and spouse.
c. Ask the person questions about the client to verify identification.
d. Give out no information about the client.

98. The best method of sharing data with staff about the positive outcomes of case management is by providing:

a. Raw data.
b. Percentages.
c. Charts and graphs.
d. Narrative explanations.

99. If the case manager contacts the pharmacist regarding a client's medications and verifies the prescriptions with the physician, this meets the case management goal of:

a. Coordinating care.
b. Improving the quality of care.
c. Encouraging client engagement.
d. Reducing health care costs.

100. The client who has been covered by an employer-sponsored insurance plan but is not qualified to apply for COBRA is a:

a. Client who was laid off from work.
b. Client who divorced the primary insurance holder (employee).
c. Client who was terminated from the job that provided the insurance due to gross misconduct.
d. Widow/Widower of the deceased primary insurance holder.

101. A pharmacy benefit manager (PBM) is primarily responsible for:

a. Providing prescription drug plans.
b. Administering prescription drug plans.
c. Assisting clients to obtain necessary drugs.
d. Preventing abuse of drugs.

102. Most medical insurance will not cover:

a. Hospice care.
b. Skilled nursing care.
c. Sub-acute care.
d. Intermediate care.

103. A client who qualified for 18 months of COBRA coverage as a beneficiary and was determined by Social Security to be disabled 40 days after beginning coverage and remained disabled for the entire 18 months is entitled to a total of:

a. 18 months of coverage.
b. 29 months of coverage.
c. 36 months of coverage.
d. 48 months of coverage.

104. The case manager working with clients with substance abuse usually focuses on assisting clients to:

a. Benefit from therapy.
b. Obtain needed resources.
c. Develop motivation for change.
d. Avoid hospitalization.

105. When transferring a client from a bed to a chair, the proper transfer technique to use with a cooperative client able to bear only partial weight and having almost no upper body strength is:

a. Stand and pivot technique.
b. Powered standing assist with 1 caregiver.
c. Seated transfer aid.
d. Full body sling lift with 2 caregivers.

106. The primary determinant as to whether people enroll in employer-sponsored health coverage is the:

a. Wages of the applicant.
b. Cost to the applicant.
c. Age of applicant.
d. Ethnicity and gender of applicant.

107. The percentage of employees who are employed in businesses that offer insurance is the:

a. Offer rate.
b. Enrollment-when-eligible rate.
c. Enrollment rate.
d. Eligibility rate.

108. If an insurance company has denied coverage for therapy that the case manager feels should have been covered for a client, the first thing the case manager should do is:

a. Determine an alternative.
b. Assist the client to file an appeal.
c. Ask the physician to call the insurance company.
d. Call the insurance company directly.

109. When evaluating research, the *P* value that is most statistically significant is:

a. 0.01
b. 0.5
c. 0.002
d. 0.04

110. Clients who are receiving physical therapy as part of community rehabilitation through a home health agency and Medicare can expect to receive:

a. 1 to 3 hours of therapy, usually 5 days a week.
b. 30 minutes to 1 hour of therapy, usually 3 days a week.
c. 3 hours of therapy, usually 3 days a week.
d. 3 or more hours of therapy, usually 5 days a week.

111. The situation that is not covered by the Family and Medical Leave Act is:

a. The client's spouse wants family leave to care for the client during a short-term illness.
b. The client wants medical leave because of a high-risk pregnancy.
c. The client wants medical leave because of cancer treatment.
d. A sibling wants family leave to care for the client during a serious illness.

112. The factor that has the most significant effect on hospital length of stay is:

a. Age.
b. Comorbidities.
c. Number of surgical procedures.
d. Diagnosis.

113. If a caregiver keeps a client with moderate dementia heavily sedated so that the client sleeps most of the day, this is an example of:

a. A safety measure.
b. Neglect.
c. Psychological abuse.
d. Physical abuse.

114. If a client with COPD has tried repeatedly to quit smoking but feels that quitting is impossible, the case manager should:

a. Remind the client of the health benefits of smoking cessation.
b. Provide support and assist the client in establishing short- and long-term goals.
c. Remind the client of the adverse effects of smoking.
d. Enlist family member is pressuring the client to quit.

115. A client who suffers from posttraumatic stress syndrome, which interferes with his ability to work and communicate with others, would be best classified as having:

a. Mental impairment.
b. Psychiatric disability.
c. Psychiatric illness.
d. Psychological illness.

116. The purpose of health coaching is to:

a. Teach clients about their diseases.
b. Help clients achieve their goals.
c. Teach clients about preventive measures.
d. Help clients understand their insurance plans.

117. A client's case management plan should focus on:

a. Determining needed resources.
b. Establishing goals and prioritizing needs.
c. Identifying strategies for care and interventions.
d. Providing cost-effective care.

118. A situation that requires termination of case management includes:

a. The client is uncooperative with case management plan.
b. The client has met maximum allowable benefit for case management.
c. The client's cost of care exceeds that projected.
d. The client has failed to meet goals and expected outcomes.

119. Before receiving benefits, the client with a preferred provider organization (PPO) insurance plan may have to pay:

a. A copayment.
b. The deductible.
c. The premium only.
d. The deductible and a copayment.

120. The agency that provides guidelines and staff training for case managers related to transitions of care is:

a. Commission on Accreditation of Rehabilitation Facilities (CARF).
b. Utilization Review Accreditation Commission (URAC).
c. American Institute of Outcomes Care Management (AIOCM).
d. Agency for Healthcare Research and Quality (AHRQ).

121. A warning sign that a case manager is developing a relationship with a client that is too personal is the case manager:

a. Enjoying meeting with the client.
b. Recognizing that the client's values are different from the case manager's.
c. Feeling attracted to a client but not acting on the attraction.
d. Asking the client about personal matters unrelated to the client's needs.

122. When conducting an interview, the case manager should avoid questions that begin with:

a. Why.
b. When.
c. Where.
d. How.

123. An indigent uninsured client with a medical emergency must be provided care at:

a. Any private physician's office.
b. Any emergency department.
c. Any public hospital.
d. Free clinics only.

124. When a client's condition does not progress according to expectations as outlined in the clinical pathway, this is referred to as a(n):

a. Variance.
b. Complication.
c. Error.
d. Discrepancy.

125. The primary function of the case manager is:

a. Coordination of care.
b. Quality management.
c. Cost management.
d. Outcomes management.

126. The primary goal of community-based case management is:

a. Assist clients to meet personal goals.
b. Coordinate services to ensure optimal outcomes and prevent hospitalization.
c. Assist clients to access services to promote independent functioning.
d. Provide care in the most cost-effective manner.

127. An appropriate statement for a case manager to make on a social networking site about working with clients is:

a. "I really like some of my clients, especially the older woman who calls me 'dear.'"
b. "I had a client today who threw a screaming fit at me."
c. "I have to see way too many clients in a day!"
d. No statement whatsoever.

128. *Sentinel procedures* refers to:

a. Procedures that resulted in a client's death.
b. Procedures associated with life-threatening diseases/conditions.
c. First procedures carried out on a client.
d. Procedures that place the client at risk of complications.

129. When doing financial analysis of diagnosis-related groups (DRGs), *relative weights* refer to value assigned to DRG based on:

a. Diagnoses only.
b. Complexity and resources needed.
c. Estimated length of stay.
d. Level of care and diagnoses.

130. A client who is temporarily disabled and has short-term disability insurance should usually expect to collect:

a. 100% of pre-disability salary.
b. 75% of pre-disability salary.
c. 60% of pre-disability salary.
d. 50% of pre-disability salary.

131. In order to consult effectively with a client and family about client needs, the first step is to:

a. Outline possible interventions.
b. Establish a trusting relationship.
c. Identify desired outcomes.
d. Evaluate the client's/family's resources.

132. The term that refers to a case manager's area of practice or knowledge is:

a. Function.
b. Role.
c. Venue.
d. Domain.

133. In motivational interviewing, *change talk* refers to:

a. Instructions provided by the interviewer.
b. A statement of goals by the client.
c. Statements indicating commitment to change.
d. A summarizing statement of client's progress.

134. A client who refuses to talk to the case manager because her husband had a bad experience with a case manager is exhibiting a barrier to communication involving:

a. Physical interference.
b. Impaired processing ability.
c. Psychological impairment.
d. Perceptions.

135. If a client has not been adhering to the plan of care, the best solution for the case manager is to:

a. Discontinue case management services.
b. Notify the client's physician.
c. Discuss barriers to adherence with the client.
d. Remind the client of his or her responsibilities.

136. When doing telephonic case management, the primary focus is usually on:

a. Cost-effective use of resources.
b. Answering questions.
c. Triaging clients.
d. Authorizing services.

137. If the case manager is concerned that a client's attention seems to wander, the best test to assess attention is:

a. Confusion Assessment Method.
b. Time and Change Tool.
c. Digit Repetition Test.
d. Trail Making Test.

138. The case manager may break a client's confidentiality:

a. Under no circumstances.
b. When a client is in need of emergent care.
c. When the client fails to follow the case management plan.
d. When the client fails to keep an appointment.

139. A bipolar client who is very nervous about transitioning into the community from a sheltered environment may benefit from:

a. A support group.
b. A 12-step program.
c. Antidepressants.
d. Peer counseling.

140. According to the Americans with Disabilities Act (ADA), public transportation must provide lifts that can accommodate occupied manual or powered wheelchairs that weigh up to a minimum of:

a. 500 pounds.
b. 600 pounds.
c. 700 pounds.
d. 800 pounds.

141. A client who insists that the case manager sit down with the client and explain the health care options in detail and outline them in writing is exhibiting:

a. Anxiety.
b. Arrogance.
c. Self-determination.
d. Self-advocacy.

142. To increase compliance, the case manager who institutes changes in procedures in order to improve patient outcomes should include:

a. Penalties.
b. Supervision.
c. Accountability.
d. Raw supportive data.

143. The primary purpose of predictive modeling is to:

a. Develop an effective model of care.
b. Predict hospital length-of-stay and need for care.
c. Increase cost-effectiveness of client care.
d. Identify clients at risk for negative outcomes.

144. A core indicator of end-stage disease is:

a. Serum albumin <2.5 g/dL.
b. Difficulty swallowing.
c. Increased medical complications.
d. Significant dyspnea, even with oxygen.

145. A hospice case manager is primarily responsible for:

a. Providing emotional support to the dying and family members.
b. Ensuring that costs related to care are minimized.
c. Ensuring dying clients remain in their home rather than in a hospital.
d. Coordinating services to provide care and comfort to the dying.

146. The primary goal of a work hardening program is for the client to:

a. Increase strength and mobility.
b. Evaluate the need for job modifications.
c. Return to full work.
d. Determine the degree to which a client can return to work.

147. If conducting a behavioral health assessment for a client who is noncompliant with treatment, the case manager should focus on:

a. Behavior in the home.
b. Behavior outside the home (work, social gatherings).
c. The effects of behavior.
d. The reason for behavior.

148. Under Medicare A's inpatient prospective payment system, the organization should expect to be paid according to the payment classification of:

a. Medicare severity diagnosis-related group (MS-DRG).
b. Fee-for-service (FFS).
c. Case-mix group (CMG).
d. Ambulatory payment category (APC).

149. When clients have multiple comorbidities and are under the care of multiple physicians, one of the first things the case manager should assess is:

a. Financial condition.
b. Psychological status.
c. Medication reconciliation.
d. Functional ability.

150. Clients with schizophrenia, depression, or bipolar disease are at high risk for:

a. Violent behavior.
b. Impaired mobility.
c. Seizure disorders.
d. Dual diagnosis.

151. The case manager should always avoid:

a. Working extended hours with one client.
b. Dual relationships with clients.
c. Working in more than one role.
d. Empathizing with clients about their conditions.

152. Self-directed Medicaid services allows participants to:

a. Make decisions about all aspects of services.
b. Apply for Medicaid services over the Internet.
c. Determine how much financial support they need.
d. Make decisions over certain specified services.

153. In utilization management, an example of misutilization is:

a. Inappropriate admission.
b. Inadequate diagnostic testing.
c. Inappropriate length of stay.
d. Treatment error.

154. A verbal exchange with a client should be documented as:

a. "Client angry and uncooperative."
b. "Client states treatment is not working and, therefore, refused to take medications."
c. "Client refusing treatment, including medications."
d. "Client appears upset with the medical care received."

155. The case manager realizes that when a client transitions between providers, the client is:

a. At increased risk for complications and negative outcomes.
b. Likely to show continued improvement and less need for care.
c. Likely to have decreased information and participation in care.
d. More likely to ask that case management be discontinued.

156. For a client covered by Medicare A for rehabilitation hospitalization, the admission functional independence measure (FIM) scores must be obtained during the first:

a. 24 hours.
b. 48 hours.
c. 3 calendar days.
d. 5 calendar days.

157. According to the Rancho Los Amigos Levels of Cognitive Functioning tool, a client with a score of VIII is:

a. Nonresponsive to all types of stimuli.
b. Confused and agitated.
c. Exhibiting a localized response to stimuli.
d. Exhibiting appropriate behavior.

158. The primary goal of quality improvement projects is to:

a. Evaluate where and how medical errors occur.
b. Assign blame for medical errors.
c. Determine the need for improvement.
d. Develop cost-saving processes.

159. If an uninsured client who is ineligible for Medicaid is unable to pay for an expensive chemotherapeutic drug, the initial step to solving the problem is to:

a. Suggest the client ask the physician about taking a less expensive drug.
b. Contact the physician to ask if the client can be treated without charge.
c. Suggest the client conduct a fund-raising campaign.
d. Determine if the drug company has a pharmaceutical assistance program.

160. Generally, the most important factor in whether a purchaser profits from a viatical settlement is the:

a. Length of time the insured lives after purchase.
b. Original purchase price of the plan.
c. Monthly payment schedule for the plan.
d. Face value of the plan on payment of benefits.

161. In order to meet the recent work test for Social Security Disability Insurance (SSDI), a client who becomes disabled in the quarter when he turns 30 years old must have worked:

a. 1.5 years out of the previous 3-year period.
b. 3 years out of the previous 5-year period.
c. 4.5 years out of previous 9-year period.
d. 5 years out of the previous 10-year period.

162. When conducting a client needs assessment as part of caseload calculations, the most important factors are:

a. Acuity, personal/family psychosocial issues, and environment.
b. Diagnosis, personal psychosocial issues, and length of stay.
c. Acuity, age, and environment.
d. Diagnosis, mental status, and functional ability.

163. With the accelerated rapid-cycle change approach to quality improvement, the team members focus on:

a. Analysis.
b. Solutions.
c. Problems.
d. Work flow.

164. Health insurance is based on the principle of:

a. Risk management.
b. Risk reduction.
c. Risk avoidance.
d. Risk pooling.

165. A client covered by the Civilian Health and Medical Program of the Department of Veterans Affairs (CHAMPVA) would need preauthorization for:

a. Durable medical equipment (purchase cost of $1,000 or more).
b. Referral to specialists.
c. Diagnostic procedures.
d. Hospice services.

166. According to Tuckman's stages of group development, the stage in which differences of opinion come to the surface and members begin forming subgroups with those who share similar opinions is:

a. Storming.
b. Norming.
c. Performing.
d. Mourning.

167. If a client with a disability is applying for a job and asks the case manager if he should disclose the disability to the employer, the best response is:

a. "It's always best to disclose a disability."
b. "You only need to disclose if you expect an accommodation."
c. "It's best to never disclose unless asked directly."
d. "Whatever you feel comfortable doing is fine."

168. Resource utilization groups (RUGs) and minimum data sets (MDSs) are used to establish payment rates for:

a. Home health agencies.
b. Ambulatory client care.
c. Acute care hospitals.
d. Skilled nursing facilities.

169. If the case manager is utilizing video calls with clients rather than in-person visits, the HIPAA regulations regarding privacy and security:

a. Must apply.
b. Are less stringent.
c. Can be waived.
d. Do not apply.

170. According to the Transtheoretical Model of change, the process of change that people go through when they express feelings (positive and negative) about change is:

a. Self-liberation.
b. Dramatic relief.
c. Consciousness raising.
d. Self-reevaluation.

171. In order to qualify for inpatient rehabilitation, a client must be able to undergo rehabilitation therapy for:

a. At least 3 hours daily for 5 to 7 days per week.
b. Less than 3 hours daily for up to 5 days per week.
c. 1 hour of therapy 5 days per week.
d. At least 5 hours of therapy 5 days per week.

172. An example of an appropriate documentation for a client who appears inebriated during a face-to-face visit is:

a. "Client appears very inebriated."
b. "Client unsteady and speech slurred from drinking."
c. "Client unsteady on feet, speech is slurred, and smells of alcohol."
d. "Client needed to reschedule visit."

173. In the Patient-Centered Medical Home Model of care, the team leader coordinating care is usually a:

a. Case manager.
b. Nurse.
c. Social worker.
d. Physician.

174. The most common strategy used to contain pharmaceutical costs is:

a. Use of generic drugs.
b. Use of preferred drug lists.
c. Volume purchasing of drugs.
d. Use of mail order prescriptions.

175. The most important factor in cost management is:

a. Purchasing in bulk and limiting choices in equipment and supplies.
b. Conducting cost comparisons and choosing the least expensive options.
c. Providing the minimal care necessary to achieve acceptable outcomes.
d. Eliminating duplication of services and care fragmentation.

176. *Failure to rescue* refers to:

a. Inability to identify life-threatening complications in time to prevent death.
b. Failure to identify clients in abusive situations.
c. Failure to prevent death in clients who experienced severe trauma.
d. Inability to prevent a client from experiencing a psychotic break.

177. The Chronic Care Model is primarily utilized in the:

a. Client's home.
b. Primary care setting.
c. Skilled nursing facility.
d. Acute hospital.

178. The purpose of the Patient Activation Measure (PAM) is to:

a. Assess client's health status.
b. Assess client's ability for self-care.
c. Identify clients who require interventions.
d. Determine client's readiness for learning.

179. A case manager who influences members of a group but is not in turn influenced by the members is exemplifying:

a. Sequential interdependence.
b. Mutual, reciprocal interdependence.
c. Unilateral interdependence.
d. Multilevel interdependence.

180. In order to qualify for Supplemental Security Income (SSI), the maximum limit for resources for a married couple is:

a. $1,000.
b. $2,500.
c. $3,000.
d. $4,000.

Answer Key and Explanations for Test #2

1. A: While regulations vary somewhat from state to state, generally assisted living facilities must have 24-hour staffing to assist clients with ADLs, housekeeping, recreation, transportation, and medication management, but skilled nursing care is not required. Different types of assisted living facilities include group homes, adult foster care, residential care facilities, and sheltered housing. Assisted living facilities or care may be provided in continuing-care communities in which clients may first live independently, before they move to an area that provides assisted care as the need arises.

2. B: A situation that may be perceived as a conflict of interest is if the case manager refers clients to a physical therapy practice run by the case manager's brother-in-law. If the brother-in-law's practice is listed along with other local practices, this is generally acceptable as long as the case manager does not try to influence the client's decision. Asking that a client be assigned to a different case manager when there is a conflict of interest, such as knowing the client well, is the appropriate action.

3. A: The most useful way in which to divide groups of clients is by risk stratification. Once the case manager has established groups of clients in similar situations, then the groups are divided by risk stratification (usually through a software program) into those at low risk, medium risk, and high risk so that the case manager can focus efforts on those with the greatest need. In any large group of clients, usually about 20% are at high risk and will need more resources.

4. C: If a $100,000 investment in hiring a case manager results in savings of $120,000, then $20,000 represents the return on investment (ROI). With ROI, the returns may be in the form of profit or savings, although savings may be more difficult to calculate with accuracy. ROI is calculated for a specific period of time, usually 1 year.

5. B: The average length of stay in an acute care hospital for a client at least 65 years of age with septicemia ranges from approximately 8 to 10 days, depending on the age and gender, with those older than 85 years having slightly shorter lengths of stay than those younger than 85. Average length of stay is determined by dividing the days of acute care by the number of discharges based on a sampling of clients with diagnoses based on the International Classification of Disease.

6. B: If the client chooses to forego transfer to an inpatient rehabilitation center and have home health care instead against the advice of the physician and the case manager, and the case manager alters the plan of care to correspond with the client's wishes, the case manager is exhibiting the ethical principle of autonomy. The case manager is respecting the client's wishes and doing what the client feels is best while respecting the right of the client to exercise autonomy.

7. A: In dealing with conflict, a staff person who follows the guidelines of the case manager he or she disagrees with is exhibiting accommodation, which is cooperative but nonassertive. Other modes of dealing with conflict include competing, collaborating, compromising, and avoiding. Competing and collaborating are assertive while avoiding and accommodating are unassertive behaviors. Avoiding and competing are uncooperative while collaborating and accommodating are cooperative. Compromising is the middle ground between asserting and cooperating and between competing and accommodating.

8. A: If a case manager works with a second case manager and has observed the second case manager falsifying records of contacts that the second case manager did not actually make, the correct action is to immediately report the situation to the supervisor/employer. A case manager has a duty to report the negligence of a coworker. By failing to make the required contacts, the second case manager is providing negligent care and making fraudulent claims about it.

9. D: If a client was seriously injured at work but feel that the employer was negligent and plans to sue, the client should file suit and avoid applying for workers' compensation because workers' compensation regulations require that the individual that receives benefits relinquish the right to sue for negligence. Workers' compensation is a state-run program that may vary somewhat from one state to another but is an insurance policy to cover wages and medical care for those injured at work.

10. B: When completing a cost-benefit analysis, an example of a "soft" cost savings is prevention of complications. Soft cost savings refer to those costs that are avoided and are difficult to calculate directly based on one patient, but may be calculated over time by looking at multiple patients and historical costs. "Hard" savings are those that relate directly to actions taken by the case manager, such as decreased length of hospitalization stay, client's change to a provider in the network, and transfer from an acute level of care to a lower level of care.

11. A: Prior to the initial interview with a client, the case manager should review the client's medical records, including both current records and records of previous hospitalization or care. The case manager should make an appointment and tell the client whom the case manager represents (hospital, insurance company) and how long the appointment should take. The case manager should introduce himself/herself to the client and take time to establish rapport with the client before beginning the formal interview and assessment. The case manager should summarize findings and discuss the plan of care at the end of the interview.

12. C: If a client in an acute care hospital is stable but will require 7 further days of IV antibiotics during recovery from surgery and a severe post-operative infection, the most appropriate level of care is a subacute care facility. Subacute facilities are sometimes stand-alone facilities or a special unit in an acute care hospital. Subacute care is intended for clients who are stable but still have a need for ongoing in-patient care for a limited period of time.

13. C: Under the hospice benefit for end-of-life care, *home* is defined as any place the client is residing, and this can include jail, residential care facilities, primary residences, or licensed health care facilities. The aim of hospice care is to provide comfort care in the "home" environment with support for not only the client but also family members and caregivers. Hospice provides services needed to maintain the client in the home, including home health aide, social services, durable medical equipment, pain medication, and medical supplies.

14. D: Passive acquisition of cases refers to acquisition by referral from health care providers, such as from physicians or nursing staff who determine a client is in need of case management, often based on a change in the client's diagnosis or condition that results in increased need for services. This type of acquisition of clients is becoming more common as health care providers become more familiar with the services the case manager provides, especially when the case manager is an active member of a team.

15. D: Temporary total disability (TTD) is paid for the time period when a person is unable to work. Temporary partial disability is paid when a person is able to work part-time but cannot yet resume full-time work. Permanent partial impairment is paid as an addition to regular disability payments if the person has a permanent disability of some type related to the injury, such as amputation of a finger. Permanent total disability is paid when the person is too disabled as a result of the injury to earn a regular income.

16. D: Under Health Insurance Portability and Accountability Act (HIPAA) regulations, clients who request copies of laboratory results or other medical records must generally receive them within 30 days. A client or client designee may request laboratory results from the physician or directly from the laboratory. The request may have to be submitted in writing, and the client or client's designee may have to pay any costs, such as for CDs, copying, and mailing.

17. A: A discharge planning evaluation must include an evaluation of the client's need for post-hospitalization services and the availability of those services. The client must also be evaluated for the ability to manage self-care and to be cared for within the environment from which the client was initially admitted. Clients should be assessed on admission to determine the need for discharge planning. These clients should include all those at risk for adverse effects after discharge in the absence of discharge planning.

18. A: The CMS Clinical Quality Measures, in their Adult Recommended Core Measures, recommend that screening for depression (NQF 0418) begin at age 12. Other core measure includes controlling hypertension, avoiding high-risk medications in elderly patients, screening and cessation intervention for tobacco use, use of imaging for low back pain, documenting current medications, BMI screening and follow-up, receiving a specialist report, and completing functional status assessment.

19. B: If a client on Medicare requires durable medical equipment, the costs should be covered by Medicare B, which also covers outpatient services, diagnostic tests, and home health care. Medicare A covers inpatient services, such as hospitalization, including different levels from acute to skilled nursing facilities and hospice and rehabilitation care. Medicare C covers services normally covered by Medicare A and B for Medicare Advantage plans. Medicare D is the prescription drug plan.

20. D: An emergent group is one that emerges as a result of mutual interest over time, and can include a group of friends. In a work environment, this type of emergent group usually does not have specific goals, unlike planned groups, but can influence attitudes. Emergent groups do not have explicit rules but an unstated understanding of the behavior that is consistent with the group norm. The group boundaries tend to be more fluid than in planned groups, so members may come and go.

21. A: Focused utilization management programs that target only specific client populations often result in cost savings and improved care. Cost savings are derived from limiting the scope of utilization management so it requires fewer staff hours as well as from better provision of care resulting from the process. Utilization management, for example, may focus on high-risk or chronic care clients, areas in which early intervention and appropriate referrals and coordination of care have the potential to improve client outcomes.

22. A: The National Quality Forum's CMS readmission measures cover heart attack, heart failure, pneumonia, COPD and knee/hip replacement, but do not cover pulmonary embolism. NQF is focusing on reducing readmissions by 10% as a means to improve client care and outcomes and to reduce costs through its All-Cause Admissions and Readmissions Measures project. Studies indicate that approximately 20% of Medicare clients are readmitted to a hospital within 30 days of discharge.

23. B: An indemnity insurance plan is usually a fee-for-service type plan. This type of plan may include a deductible and a copayment, which may vary depending on the cost and type of plan. Fee-for-service plans usually allow clients to choose their physicians, although clients may be limited by the physicians available. The types of preventive services available to clients will also vary. Preventive services are usually exempt from the deductible and may or may not require copayment.

24. B: If a client was injured at work and is undergoing rehabilitation for physical strengthening 2 days a week in preparation for returning to work, this is referred to as work conditioning. Work hardening is more intensive and involves rehabilitation for 3 to 5 days a week. Work adjustment focuses on the skills and abilities the client will need to be successful at work. Some clients return to the job with transitional work duty; that is, the work load has been modified to fit the ability of the client.

25. A: When the client of a mental health case manager refuses case management after being discharged from a mental institution, the case manager should assess the need for court-ordered case management by determining if the client appears to pose a threat to self or others. The case manager must consider the patient's history, diagnosis, and circumstances of admission to the facility and discharge, as well as the client's compliance with treatment and potential for growth.

26. C: A swing bed agreement with CMS allows a hospital to use the same bed for acute or skilled nursing facility (SNF) care, depending on the needs of the client. This agreement is used primarily for small or rural facilities where alternate types of facilities offering different levels of care are not readily available in the community. Clients may be admitted into acute care and transitioned to SNF care while staying in the same room and bed, although the level of care that they receive will be different.

27. D: When doing case management evaluation using the cost-effectiveness analysis method, *sensitivity analysis* refers to testing assumptions and validating conclusions in order to determine if there are alternate explanations that could explain costs and benefits. The cost-effectiveness analysis method includes 6 principles: (1) statement of analytic perspective, (2) description of anticipated benefits, (3) outline of types of costs, (4) adjustment for differential timing (discounting), (5) sensitivity analysis, and (6) summary of measurement of efficiency (cost-effectiveness ratio).

28. D: If a client's insurance is an exclusive provider organization (EPO) and the client chooses to see a physician outside of the network and receives a bill for $500, the client must pay 100%. With an EPO, there is no gatekeeper physician, so the client is able to make an appointment with a specialist without a referral, but the program limits coverage to those physicians who are contracted with the EPO except in the case of emergency. However, even with an emergency, once the client is stabilized, the client should be transferred to the care of physicians in the EPO, and this may require transfer to a different hospital.

29. B: For payer-based case management services, contact with the client is usually via telephone. Payer-based case managers are usually located at insurance companies or work from their homes rather than in the community or in healthcare facilities, so they typically have little direct contact with clients. Case managers may be contacted directly by a client or the client's family or support person, or they may receive a referral from a healthcare provider or a member of the insurance company (such as a medical director or claims adjuster).

30. D: The Digit Repetition Test is primarily used to diagnose attention deficits in those with normal intelligence. The test requires the client to listen and repeat numbers, starting with two random single-digit numbers (such as 3, 7) and then adding a third number to a different sequence (such as 7, 4, 9) each time the client answers correctly. A normal score for a person with average intelligence is the ability to repeat 5 to 7 numbers. A score below 5 indicates impaired attention.

31. C: A terminally ill client who believes that prayer will heal her probably depends on faith for comfort. A deeply held belief in the power of prayer is common to many who are profoundly religious and does not mean the client is in denial or not dealing realistically with his or her condition. For example, Christian Scientists routinely turn to prayer to heal sickness and eschew medicine, and believe that it is God's will if they are not healed.

32. C: When a client has signed a release of information form so the case manager can provide information to a therapist or any other individual, the case manager should release the minimum information necessary to meet the request. If, for example, the request does not include the initial assessment or progress notes, then the case manager should not include those with the records released. Even when records are released, the case manager should remain aware of the client's right to confidentiality and privacy.

33. A: In order for an organization to receive health plan accreditation from the National Committee for Quality Assurance (NCQA), the organization must report measures of performance in more than 100 areas. These measures fall under 6 standards: quality management and improvement, population health management, network management, utilization management, credentialing, and member experience. Outcomes evaluation is a subset within the quality management and improvement standard. Accreditation requires a comprehensive initial review and then submission of annual reports.

34. B: A client who is a devoutly religious Catholic and believes her health problems are punishment for sins may benefit most from pastoral counseling because a priest who is trained as a therapist may help the client balance religious and health beliefs in a more realistic manner. Pastoral counselors often carry out both psychological and spiritual counseling, providing the client with the support of the faith community. Pastoral counselors may represent many different faiths and branches of religions.

35. C: The score for the REALM (Rapid Estimate of Adult Literacy in Medicine) test is based on the number of words the client can pronounce. The client is given a form with three different lists of medical terms in increasing difficulty from simple one syllable words (fat, flu, stress), to two (bowel, asthma, rectal), and to three and four (appendix, menopause, potassium, osteoporosis). The client reads the lists aloud and is allowed to skip unfamiliar words.

36. C: A Karnofsky Performance Status Scale score of 30 indicates that the client is severely disabled and unable to attend to ADLs independently and likely requires institutional or hospital care. The Karnofsky Performance Status Scale classifies clients according to their functional abilities and impairments with scores ranging from 100 (normal with no indications of disease) to 0 (death). Scores of 80 to 100 indicate the client is independent in care, 50 to 70 indicates the inability to work but the ability to live at home with some assistance at times. Scores of 10 to 40 indicate the need for institutionalization/hospitalization.

37. C: Palliative care is intended for those who need to improve their quality of life by managing symptoms. Palliative care can begin at any point during an illness and is unrelated to diagnosis or life expectancy. Unlike hospice care, palliative care clients can be undergoing curative treatments. Many clients with life-threatening diseases or chronic illnesses may begin with palliative care for control of pain or other symptoms and then may progress to hospice care as their condition deteriorates and they opt to have no further curative treatments.

38. A: The case manager who wants to justify further intervention for a rehabilitation client who has not met performance goals should begin with the data on admission to the program. For example, if one of the goals is the ability to walk up 2 flights of stairs, the beginning data may include the ability to walk up and down 3 steps. This should be followed by the current data, such as the ability to walk up one flight of stairs. Then, the case manager should outline the goal and any pertinent information.

39. C: When considering whether the Americans with Disabilities Act will provide protections for a client, the case manager recognizes that a condition that may be considered a disability is alcoholism. An employer can require that employees not be under the influence of alcohol and prohibit the presence or intake of alcohol in the workplace, as well as discipline or discharge an employee whose alcohol usage negatively impacts job performance. However, if an individual's alcoholism substantially impairs major life activities, it can be ruled as a disability. Compulsive gambling, pyromania, and kleptomania are all specifically excluded by the A.D.A.

40. D: In a payer-based case management model, the case manager is generally an employee of the insurance company and must ensure that the client receives competent and quality care while still ensuring that the care is cost-effective. Payer-based case management may present the case manager with ethical dilemmas because the insurance company may be more focused on cost-effectiveness than client needs; however, the case manager must retain the role of client advocate and try to balance concerns.

41. D: The purpose of admission certification is to determine the medical necessity of admission to a hospital or other health care institution. Admission certification is a form of utilization management that is carried out prior to admission to ensure clients will get the appropriate level of care and usually includes estimates of length of stay for the client's diagnosis. Admission certification is not a determination of benefits, so it does not guarantee care will be paid for.

42. C: The FOCUS performance improvement model to facilitate change is primarily used to identify problems. The model is usually used in conjunction with other change models (such as PDCA) to find solutions to the problems. FOCUS:

- *Find*: Review the organization for processes that aren't working well (problems).
- *Organize*: Create a team with people who understand the problem.
- *Clarify*: Use brainstorming to find solutions.
- *Uncover*: Determine the reason the problem has occurred.
- *Start*: Begin the change process.

43. A: The most common reasons for screening clients to determine need for case management are diagnosis, high rates of resource utilization (often exemplified by repeat or frequent hospitalizations and visits to the emergency department), and high costs of care in dollar amounts (usually within a set duration of time, such as the preceding 6 to 12 months). This type of screening is often automated so that these clients are tagged on admission and referred to case management. This may exclude some clients whose diagnosis and/or condition changes after admission.

44. B: When preparing a quality improvement report, the case manager should begin by identifying the indicator that was measured (such as length of stay for myocardial infarction), providing any necessary background information or historical statistics. Then, the case manager should outline interventions utilized to bring about improvement. The case manager should explain the type of measurement used for assessment and the final results of that assessment. The results may be presented in various formats, but visual formats (charts, graphs) are usually the easiest for staff to interpret.

45. C: Physical disability: Defect in body function, such as may occur with chronic conditions, such as osteoarthritis in the knees. Sensory disability: Vision and hearing deficits as well as impaired sense of taste and smell, touch, and balance. Intellectual disability: Cognitive impairment, fragile X syndrome. Mental disability: Mental health disorder that impairs functioning. Pervasive developmental disability: Impaired ability to socialize and communicate, such as with autism. Developmental disability: Impaired growth and development, such as with spina bifida.

46. B: In an acute care hospital interdisciplinary team, the individual primarily responsible for assessing the post-discharge needs of the client is the case manager. While all members of the team collaborate to provide care within the acute care hospital and some may be actively involved in planning for post-discharge needs, the responsibility still remains with the case manager who must not only identify needs but determine the community resources available to meet those needs and make arrangements for necessary community providers.

47. A: To prevent back injury, items to be lifted should be 30 to 40 inches above the floor or the surface the person is standing on. In some cases, people may need to stand on a stool, or table height may need to be lowered. If reaching for items on shelves, the person should use a stepstool or portable steps, making sure that the equipment is appropriate. Work surfaces that are of variable height are ideal but not always available.

48. C: The purpose of a concurrent review (also known as continued stay review) of a hospitalized client is to assess the client's need for continued hospitalization as well as to assess the client's level of care. For example, a client may be assessed to determine if continued ICU care is necessary or if the client can be moved to a primary care unit. This type of review is done on an ongoing, often daily, basis during the client's hospitalization.

49. A: In Robert's Seven-Stage Crisis Intervention Model, the first stage includes assessing lethality and the potential for danger. Seven stages include:

5. Psychosocial/Lethality assessment
6. Rapid establishment of rapport by showing respect, making eye contact, and being positive
7. Identify major problems/precipitants and prioritize, discussing client's current coping mechanisms
8. Deal with feelings/emotions, encouraging client to vent and using therapeutic communication
9. Generate and explore alternatives, collaboratively with client
10. Implement plan of action
11. Follow-up/Evaluation

50. B: The independent practice association (IPA) HMO model allows individual or groups of physicians to contract with an HMO to provide services while the physicians are also seeing non-HMO clients. The physicians maintain private practices and contract to serve clients enrolled in the HMO. In the staff model, physicians are hired by and work directly for the HMO. In the group practice model, the HMO has a contract with a large multi-specialty group that primarily sees HMO clients. With the direct contract model, the HMO contracts directly with a physician to provide services, and there is no insurer.

51. A: The best response to a client who is progressing well after a stroke (or any illness/injury) but remains extremely fearful and anxious about discharge is to explore the client's concerns with the client, allowing the client to express his or her feelings. The person may have valid reasons for concerns, such as living alone or lack of transportation, and may not fully understand the services that are available in the community or may feel overwhelmed by changes in physical condition and abilities.

52. B: RotaCare clinics are supported by health care volunteers and Rotary Clubs and provide free medical care to the uninsured, underinsured, and homeless. The clinics are located throughout the United States and treat clients with minor illnesses and injuries. Some clinics also have specialty clinics with a range of different specialists, such as dermatologists or psychiatrists, while others have lists of physicians and dentists willing to provide *pro bono* care for clients. Some clinics provide vaccinations and HIV testing as well as wellness programs and health education.

53. B: The primary purpose of a benchmark study is to compare an organization's performance against best practices of the industry to identify gaps in performance. Benchmark studies usually focus on specific processes or services and help to develop methods to adapt best practices to the workplace in order to improve performance. Benchmark studies may focus on clinical (such as outcomes of care), financial (such as cost-effectiveness, length of stay), or operational (such as the case management system in place) issues.

54. A: An elderly low-income home care client who is losing weight because she doesn't like to cook and lives on junk food may benefit most from meal delivery services, as her diet is the immediate problem. Home meal delivery services (such as Meals on Wheels) are usually reasonably priced and provide food for one to three meals daily, depending on the specific program. Assisted living facilities and homemaker services may be too expensive for a low-income client and are not usually covered by Medicare or insurance companies.

55. B: Insurance companies hire case managers primarily to reduce the costs of care. This does not mean that care is less than optimal but that the care that is provided is appropriate for the client's needs. This may mean that clients are transferred to a different level of care rather than staying in an acute care hospital or are referred to a home health agency and discharged if care can be provided at a lower cost in the home environment.

56. D: Standards of practice include statements that outline the level of performance expected of a professional, such as a case manager. The standards of practice are usually developed by professional organizations, especially those that provide certification. Case management plans outline client care procedures and expected outcomes. Standards of care outline the level of care that all clients should expect, based on evidence-based practice and outcomes data. Evidence-based practice guidelines outline care that should be provided for specific diagnoses/conditions.

57. C: The clinical resources model is the model of acute care case management that follows the client's progress through acute hospitalization to ensure effective, safe, and cost-effective transition from acute care to post-acute care. The integrated functional model refers to case management that includes the responsibility for both utilization review and discharge planning. The disease management model focuses on post-acute care for chronic diseases in order to reduce rehospitalization. The outcomes management model focuses on improving clinical outcomes and cost-effectiveness in the acute care environment.

58. C: A TRICARE beneficiary is eligible for TRICARE for Life if the person has both Medicare A and B. TRICARE for Life is a Medicare wrap-around program that allows clients to seek medical care from any Medicare provider, non-Medicare provider, military hospital, or clinic (if space is available). Claims are first paid for through Medicare and then forwarded to another healthcare provider (if available) and then to TRICARE, which will pay the balance for TRICARE-covered services.

59. C: Coverage can be 3 months retroactive (March 1) if the client would have been eligible if he or she had applied at the earlier time, allowing for coverage of medical expenses incurred prior to application. Clients are eligible for Medicaid if they are younger than 65 years and their income is up to 138% of the federal poverty level. The 100% federal poverty level (for a family of four) in 2024 was $30,000. The Affordable Care Act expanded Medicaid coverage but not all states have opted for expansion, so eligibility requirements and benefits may vary somewhat from state to state.

60. B: TRICARE Extra utilizes a paid provider organization, so the plan beneficiary receives a 5% discount on copayments. There is no additional charge for selecting this option. TRICARE provides civilian health care benefits for military, retired military, and dependents, as well as some who are in the military reserve. TRICARE is under control of the Defense Health Agency (DHA). TRICARE has a number of programs, including TRICARE for Life, which serves as a supplemental insurance to Medicare, and TRICARE Young Adult, for dependents who have aged out of TRICARE.

61. C: An individual purchasing an insurance plan through an exchange should expect that a silver tier plan will pay 70% of medical expenses. Individually purchased insurance plans are categorized by tiers, indicating the average percentage of medical expenses covered:

- Platinum: 90%
- Gold: 80%
- Silver: 70%
- Bronze: 60%

A "catastrophe" plan is also available for those under age 30 with limited income, but these plans have very limited coverage. Under the Affordable Care Act, insurance plans must cover Essential Health Benefits (EHBs).

62. D: Under Medicare Part A and/or Part B, the home health services that are covered include intermittent skilled nursing care, pathology services (lab testing), occupational therapy, respiratory therapy, physical therapy, and speech-language therapy. Medicare may also cover social services, intermittent home health aide services, and the cost of medical supplies and durable medical equipment. Services that are not covered include homemaker services, round-the-clock care, and home delivery of meals. Additionally, clients must meet specific criteria, such as being homebound and requiring intermittent skilled nursing care (for other than drawing of blood for lab tests).

63. D: The best placement for a 24-year-old client with schizophrenia being discharged from a psychiatric institution for the first time in 4 years is likely a group home that specializes in clients with mental illness and provides medication monitoring and assistance with community services and managing a budget, cooking, and housekeeping. Clients who have spent prolonged periods in psychiatric facilities may need to spend 6 to 12 months in a group home before transitioning into less supervised living situations.

64. D: The billing code that is utilized for services such as ambulance and durable medical equipment is HCPCS-Level II. HCPCS codes are used for non-physician services. Codes comprise a letter (A, B, C, D...), which designates the category (such as E code: Durable Medical Equipment) followed by 4 numbers, which designate the specific item (such as E1130 to E1161 for different types of wheelchairs).

65. C: A series of steps in treatment based on client response and developed through scientific- and evidence-based research in order to standardize a specific type of care is referred to as an algorithm. For example, Algorithms are widely used in emergency departments to determine treatment related to advanced cardiac life support. Algorithms may incorporate a decision-tree approach to aid in choosing the correct treatment. Some states (such as Texas) are using algorithms to advise Medicaid physicians about prescribing medications, such as antipsychotics.

66. D: In order to qualify for Medicare based on a 63-year-old spouse's work record, the applicant must be at least 65 years old. The qualifying spouse must be 62 years of age or older. The applicant may also qualify based on the work record of a former spouse or deceased spouse. Those who do not qualify based on their own or their spouse's work record may pay premiums for Part A, Part B, and Part D with payment for Part A prorated according to the applicant's work record.

67. C: When making decisions about case management based on catastrophic diagnoses, diagnoses would include solid-organ transplants because the potential for costly and time-consuming complications is very high. These clients often have very high rates of utilization of resources because of the need for multiple health care providers and procedures. Other catastrophic diagnoses include HIV/AIDS, kidney failure, liver failure, traumatic brain injuries, cancer/leukemia, acute respiratory distress syndrome, respiratory distress syndrome of infancy, premature delivery, and multi-trauma cases. Patients undergoing neurological surgery also may have multiple complications.

68. A: The term that would most apply to a transgender female (biological male) who is attracted to females is lesbian. While gay might also fit, this term is more commonly used to refer to male homosexuals. For legal and descriptive purposes, a transgender female is considered the same as a biological female when considering issues such as sexual attraction. Thus, a transgender male (biological female) who is attracted to females is considered heterosexual.

69. C: A cost-containment strategy in which all clients receiving similar services or treatments from the same provider have the same payment rate is all-payer rate setting. Rates may be set by the provider or by government regulations, such as through Medicaid. The goal is to reduce the high costs of health care and reduce price competition, although the costs to the provider may increase because of the need to negotiate rates and process claims, as reimbursement schedules may vary according to diagnoses or other criteria.

70. B: While a stroke client may have the need for multiple therapists, the speech therapist is specifically trained to evaluate and provide therapy for clients with difficulty swallowing. This may include exercises as well as modifications of foods (such as thickening watery liquids). The occupational therapist may assist the client in adjusting to physical limitations and learning to perform activities of daily living. The physical therapist may help to restore strength and mobility while the nutritionist may teach the client about meal planning and dietary needs.

71. C: While grief responses vary widely and the length of bereavement varies as well, because the client is having much difficulty functioning and caring for her home and family, her grieving process is exaggerated, so she will probably benefit most from referral to a bereavement counselor who can help the client move toward a more normal grieving process. As part of counseling, the counselor may suggest that the client participate in a support group for people whose spouses have died.

72. A: General Recovery is the Milliman Care Guideline that would be appropriate for clients with complex clinical situations and diagnoses for which a specific guideline does not exist. Chronic care provides guidelines for outpatient care for 20 chronic conditions. Inpatient and surgical care provides guidelines for clients needing hospitalization and/or surgery. Ambulatory care provides guidelines for managing outpatient referrals, diagnostic procedures, rehabilitation services, and pharmaceutical utilization. Home care provides guidelines for home health care, and recovery facility care provides guidelines for admission to recovery facilities and discharge planning.

73. B: The SAFE questions to ask a client suspected of being a victim of abuse include questions about Stress/Safety, Afraid/Abused, Friends/Family, and Emergency plan:

- Stress/Safety: What are your stresses? Do you feel safe?
- Afraid/Abused: Have you or your children been afraid, threatened, or abused, physically or sexually?
- Friends/Family: Do your family and friends know about the abuse? Can you tell them or ask them for support?
- Emergency plan: Do you have resources and a place to go? Do you need help finding shelter now? Do you want to see a social worker or counselor?

74. D: The instrument that is most appropriate to assess general health and disability across all medical disciplines, including mental, neurological, and substance abuse, is World Health Organization Disability Assessment Schedule 2 (WHODAS-2), which should now be used in place of the Global Assessment of Functioning (GAF) test. WHODAS-2 has 12-item and 36-item versions as well as self-administered and interviewer-administered versions. Domains include understanding and communicating, getting around, self-care, getting along with people, life activities, and participation in society.

75. A: The primary focus of job analysis is on the specific requirements of the job. This detailed analysis may include tasks, as well as time, knowledge, and skills needed to complete tasks. Other aspects include the environment, necessary tools and equipment, and relationships. Job analysis may be used to develop training programs by identifying needs, to determine the degree of compensation for a job, to develop selection procedures, and to enact performance reviews. Job analysis may include observation, surveys, and interviews.

76. A: The case manager who cannot find food or shelter for a homeless client may receive assistance for the client from the local Salvation Army, which is a Christian denominational church with international charities. While programs vary from city to city, the Salvation Army usually has programs for the homeless in most areas and often provides meals and shelter or emergency funds. The Salvation Army runs a network of thrift stores to support rehabilitation programs for substance abuse.

77. B: A case manager assigned to a population health program (which is geared toward improving the health of a particular group) in an African American community with high rates of hypertension and diabetes should initially focus education on diet and exercise because these lifestyle changes may be most effective in helping to manage both hypertension and diabetes. Interventions may include cooking and nutrition classes, support groups (especially for weight loss and diabetes), visits to farmers' markets, walking groups, and other types of exercise.

78. C: The case manager is preparing a client to undergo a functional capacity evaluation required by the client's insurance company following injury and tells the client that the evaluation will not include motivation. The FCE focuses on the ability of the client to carry out job functions and may include lifting ability, range of motion, stamina, strength measures, ability to carry items, and other physical activities that may be required by the specific type of job.

79. A: Disease management programs are usually intended for specific populations of clients, usually those identified as at high risk because of diagnosis, complications, and history of resource utilization and high costs. Part of planning the program is to research data and identify barriers to change before implementing interventions. Often pilot programs and/or focus groups are utilized to evaluate interventions. The implemented program usually includes the use of clinical practice guidelines to promote consistency and a process to evaluate outcomes.

80. B: Case management information systems (CMISs) generally include standardized plans of care to provide treatment protocols that support best practices. CMISs help to identify resources available in order to prevent complications. The systems are able to also identify patterns, variances, and trends among past and present records. If trends are identified, then the system can provide decision support to help with planning and management of care. CMISs are especially valuable for clients with complex needs, such as those who are elderly or have chronic diseases and multiple morbidities.

81. D: If the case manager wants to apply the correct diagnostic code for outpatient services to a billing form, the case manager would utilize ICD-10-CM. ICD-10 is used for diagnoses for both inpatient and outpatient services and is consistent with DSM-V, cancer registry codes, and nursing classifications. ICD-10-PCS contains procedure codes for inpatient procedures while CPT contains codes for outpatient procedures. HCPCS-Level II codes are utilized for durable medical equipment and other services, such as ambulance, not covered by other codes. NDC is national drug codes.

82. C: A point of service plan is a structure that combines aspects of an HMO with a PPO. Clients are able to receive care from health care providers within the network or may seek treatment outside the network in some circumstances. This type of plan offers more flexibility to the client, but usually there are additional costs when a client chooses to seek treatment outside of the network. Copayments may increase and the percentage of costs covered by the plan may decrease.

83. B: In negotiating prices with an out-of-network health care provider or any other negotiating, the case manager should begin by researching prices and coming to the negotiation well prepared. Negotiations may be aggressive, with one side perceived as a winner and the other side as a loser, but this type of negotiation often impairs relationships and may negatively impact future negotiations. Negotiations may also be cooperative, with each side working together to find a mutually satisfying solution. Cooperative negotiations are usually more productive and establish better working relationships.

84. D: The focus of case management in a pre-acute environment, such as a physician's office or clinic, is often on prevention, reducing the need for costly medical interventions and hospitalization. This may include monitoring client's medications and treatments to ensure compliance, doing assessment of health risks, facilitating health screenings, as well as encouraging lifestyle changes, such as increased exercise and smoking cessation, and enrolling clients in wellness programs. The case manager may do telephone triage and monitoring and make referrals to community agencies to provide the client necessary resources.

85. C: OSHA sets and enforces regulations related to workplace safety. In health care, this encompasses bloodborne pathogens, hazardous materials and hazardous wastes, and compressed gases and air equipment. OSHA also establishes lifting limits and ergonomic guidelines to minimize the risk of injury. Compliance officers can take complaints and issue citations for those out of compliance.

86. B: When counseling a client, the statement by a case manager that is a misrepresentation of qualifications is "You don't need any more physical therapy." This determination needs to be made by a physical therapist or a physician, not a case manager who does not have expertise in this area. The case manager should use care in speaking to avoid the suggestion that he or she has authority that does not exist.

87. C: Once an organization has completed the application process and received accreditation from the Commission on Accreditation of Rehabilitation Facilities (CARF) indicating the need for improvement in case management or any other aspect, the organization must submit a Quality Improvement Plan (QIP) within 90 days. The QIP should provide a blueprint of plans for improvement or outline steps already taken to remedy the problems highlighted by CARF. CARF provides standards manuals and training to help organizations understand and prepare for accreditation.

88. C: When a client tells the case manager that her caregiver does not allow her to use the telephone or read her mail, the case manager should suspect that the client is experiencing psychological abuse. Psychological abuse may include threats, coercion, and intimidation, as well as behavior that is controlling (and often isolating), such as preventing a client access to mail or the telephone. Nurses are mandatory reporters of abuse, so any evidence of abuse should be reported to the proper authorities.

89. C: The best solution to dealing with a client who expresses extreme prejudice toward ethnic minorities and the LGBT population is to provide professional services and avoid debate. The case manager should stay focused on the needs of the client rather than the client's attitudes. Case managers often encounter ethical conflicts and clients with value systems at odds with their own, and trying to change the client's ideas is generally fruitless and just leads to conflict.

90. C: The Agency for Healthcare Research and Quality (AHRQ) provides clinical guidelines and recommendations. AHRQ maintains the National Guideline Clearinghouse (NGC), which is a database with evidence-based clinical practice guidelines. Health care professionals may submit guidelines to the NGC, which provides guidance in submission and inclusion criteria. AHRQ provides information to clients and consumers as well as health care professionals and policymakers. AHRQ also produces videos (available on YouTube through AHRQ Health TV) for clients and clinicians.

91. A: Depression is common in older adults with comorbid conditions and chronic conditions affecting the quality of life, such as cancer, diabetes, arthritis, and heart disease, with approximately 37% experiencing depression. Some medications, such as steroids, diuretics, and Parkinson disease drugs may also precipitate depression. Depression is often undiagnosed because screening for depression in older adults is often neglected. The Geriatric Depression Scale is a self-assessment tool that can be used to identify those with depression.

92. A: Clients with a BMI outside of normal parameters should have a follow-up intervention plan in place and documented. The normal parameters for those who are 18 to 64 years of age are 18.5-25, so a BMI above 25 indicates the need for intervention. Normal BMI parameters for those age 65 and older are 23-30. BMI is based on height and weight, but clients should be assessed individually because muscle mass may affect results.

93. A: The Blaylock Risk Assessment Screening Score (BRASS) is a tool used to identify older adults at risk of prolonged hospitalization. These clients are often in need of intense discharge planning, so identifying the clients early allows for the planning process to begin in order to prevent unanticipated post-discharge issues. BRASS contains 10 items related to functional status, abilities, and history. Clients receive scores for each item, with a total score of 10 indicating the need for home care resources, 11-19 indicating a need for intensive discharge planning, and more than 20 indicating at risk for placement other than at home.

94. B: The FDA will allow emergency use of a drug with filing of an Investigational New Drug (IND) exemption for one client only and only one time per institution. The client's condition must be life-threatening or extremely debilitating and with no available standard treatment. There must be insufficient time to follow protocol to gain approval from the review committee, but a report must be filed with the review committee within 5 days. Consent must be obtained from the client or client's designee prior to administration of the drug.

95. A: Allowing a person to adjust work hours to accommodate a treatment schedule is an example of job modification. The actual work stays the same, but modifications are made to allow the person to carry out the necessary tasks. In this case, the hours of work are changed to accommodate treatment. Other examples of work modification include allowing people (such as cashiers) to sit instead of stand while carrying out duties or allowing a person to work fewer hours.

96. A: The best tool to combat fear of technology and data is education. Since much of medical care is now data driven, the case manager must deal with data on a daily basis, and staff members must become used to an evidence-based focus on providing care. Staff members may require technical computer training in order to use electronic records more effectively and should become familiar with the types of data that are collected and analyzed.

97. D: The case manager should give out no information about the client and should not even acknowledge the client is at the hospital because this is a violation of the patient's right to confidentiality unless the client has given permission for his wife to receive information and a method of accurate identification, such as a password, is set up in advance. Anyone can telephone and pose as a family member to get information, so the case manager must use great care.

98. C: The best method of sharing data with staff about the positive outcomes of case management is by providing charts and graphs because they are easy to interpret and information can be gleaned very quickly. Percentages are the weakest of all statistics because they can be easily manipulated. Raw data are hard to interpret, as they require the viewer to make conclusions and sometimes do calculations. Narrative explanations are more time-consuming to the viewer and may be a useful addition to charts and graphs rather than as stand-alone presentation of data.

99. A: If the case manager contacts the pharmacist regarding a client's medications and verified the prescriptions with the physician, this meets the case management goal of coordinating care. Clients often have multiple healthcare providers (primary care physician, orthopedist, endocrinologist, cardiologist) and may be prescribing different medications and treatments without adequate information about treatments prescribed by others, so the case manager must monitor all aspects of care and coordinate with all healthcare providers.

100. C: The client who has been covered by an employer-sponsored insurance plan but is not qualified to apply for COBRA is a client was terminated from the job that covered the insurance due to gross misconduct. However, if the client had been terminated due to minor reasons, divorced the primary insurance holder, or was the spouse of a primary insurance holder who died, the client is then qualified to apply for COBRA. Coverage can continue for 18-36 months, but costs may be higher because the client has to cover the complete cost of the policy.

101. B: Pharmacy benefit managers (PBMs) are primarily responsible for administering prescription drug plans, which are provided by insurance companies (such as Blue Cross) or health care systems (such as Kaiser Hospitals). PBMs process and pay claims, maintain the formulary, and establish contracts and discount agreements with pharmacies and drug companies. Examples of PBMs include Express Scripts, United Health, and CVS Caremark. PBMs may provide networks of pharmacies to which clients can go to get drugs as well as mail-order programs that allow clients to obtain 3-month supplies of drugs.

102. D: Most medical insurance will not cover intermediate care, which is a level of care slightly more intense than custodial care. The client may require nursing supervision but does not require skilled medical care or therapy. Medical insurance also does not generally cover custodial care, although in some instances Medicaid does provide custodial care. Custodial care provides clients assistance with activities of daily living and may also include homemaking services, such as cooking and cleaning.

103. B: A COBRA beneficiary who qualifies for 18 months of COBRA coverage as a beneficiary and is determined by Social Security to be disabled within 60 days of beginning COBRA coverage and who remains disabled throughout the 18-month period of coverage is entitled to apply for an 11-month extension for a total of 29 months of coverage. If a person qualifies for an extension because of disability, all qualified beneficiaries in the family are also eligible to apply for the same extension.

104. B: The case manager working with clients with substance abuse usually focuses on assisting clients to obtain needed resources. Care for those with substance abuse is often fragmented and may be costly, so the case manager must be aware of all resources in the community, such as outpatient treatment centers and 12-step programs. Clients with substance abuse often have dual diagnoses and may need treatment for mental or medical health problems as well as substance abuse. Some may be homeless and may need information about shelters and meal programs.

105. D: The proper transfer technique to use with a cooperative client able to bear only partial weight and with almost no upper body strength is a full body sling lift with 2 caregivers. Because the client lacks upper body strength, the client is unable to assist with the transfer, so other transfer techniques put both the client and the caregiver at risk for injury. Different types of slings are available, including toileting and bathing (mesh) slings.

106. B: The primary determinant as to whether people enroll in employer-sponsored health coverage is the cost to the applicant. The higher the cost, the less likely employees are to enroll. For this reason, some companies offer a range of plans with different costs. Companies may make varying contributions to the cost of the insurance plans, ranging from 100% to 0%. Salary is another important consideration with those with higher salaries more likely to purchase insurance.

107. A: Enrollment rates associated with insurance:

- Offer: The percentage of employees who are employed in businesses that offer insurance
- Enrollment-when-eligible: The percentage of employees who meet the criteria for enrollment and actually enroll in employee-sponsored health insurance plans
- Enrollment: The percentage of all workers (eligible and non-eligible) who enroll in employee-sponsored health insurance plans offered to employees
- Eligibility: The percentage of employees who meet the criteria for eligibility to enroll

108. B: If an insurance company has denied coverage for therapy that the case manager feels should have been covered for a client, the first thing the case manager should do is assist the client to file an appeal. It is not unusual for insurance companies to deny coverage, and each company has an appeal process that should be followed. The letter of denial should provide the reason for denial, but if not, the client or client's representative should call to find out the reason so that it can be addressed in the appeal.

109. C: When evaluating research, the *P* value that is most statistically significant is 0.002. The *P* value estimates the probability that the null hypothesis will be rejected. For example, if comparing two treatments, the null hypothesis states there is no difference in outcomes, so rejecting the null hypothesis means that a difference exists. If the *P* value is <0.05, this difference is generally considered to be statistically significant. A *P* value of 0.002 would be highly significant.

110. B: Clients who are receiving physical therapy as part of community rehabilitation through a home health agency can expect to receive 30 minutes to 1 hour of therapy, usually 3 days a week per therapist. If the client is receiving therapy from multiple therapists (physical therapist, occupational therapist, speech therapist), then this time limit applies to each therapist. Under original Medicare, an episode of care comprises 60 days. In order to avoid extra costs, the client should receive therapy from a home health agency that is Medicare certified.

111. D: The situation that is not covered by the Family and Medical Leave Act is a sibling who wants family leave to care for the client during a serious illness. FMLA does not extend benefits to extended family, such as grandparents, in-laws, and siblings, only close family members, such as parents, children, and spouse. FMLA provides those who are eligible up to 12 work weeks of unpaid leave each year, during which time group health benefits must be maintained. The individual must be able to return to the same or an equivalent position after leave. If caring for a service member with serious illness or injury, 26 weeks are allowed in a single year.

112. D: The factor that has the most significant effect on hospital length of stay is the client's diagnosis, accounting for over 25% of variations in length of stay. Length of stay also increases with comorbidities and with the number of surgical procedures. Age is another important factor, as elderly patients tend to have longer hospital stays than younger clients, although this is an additive factor superimposed upon diagnosis. Clients who receive discharge planning early in their hospital stay tend to have shorter lengths of stay than clients who receive later discharge planning.

113. D: If a caregiver keeps a client with moderate dementia heavily sedated so the client sleeps most of the day, this is an example of physical abuse. While much physical abuse is more obvious, with bruises and physical injuries attesting to beating, kicking, slapping, or pinching, physical abuse also includes such behaviors as forced feeding, using unnecessary physical restraints to limit a client's mobility, and using excessive drugs to control behavior, often so that the caregiver can neglect the client and avoid providing needed care.

114. B: If a client with COPD has tried repeatedly to quit smoking but feels that quitting is impossible, the case manager should provide support and assist the client in establishing short- and long-term goals. For some clients who are very resistive to quitting, cutting back on smoking may be an initial goal, and the case manager may suggest chewing nicotine gum, sucking on hard candy, or other activity when the client feels the urge to smoke.

115. B: A client who suffers from posttraumatic stress syndrome, which interferes with his ability to work and communicate with others, would be best classified as having a psychiatric disability because the client's condition interferes with his ability to function. Although some patients stabilize and go into remission with medication and treatment, because of the erratic nature of much mental illness, many clients have a psychiatric disability and may be eligible for Social Security disability payments.

116. B: The purpose of health coaching (also referred to as wellness coaching) is to help clients achieve their goals. The case manager encourages the client to identify their own problems and set goals for change, serving as a support rather than an instructor. The primary role of the case manager is to listen and respond. The case manager helps the clients explore ways of achieving their goals and monitors their progress as they make positive changes.

117. B: A client's case management plan should focus on establishing goals and prioritizing needs. The plan is developed from the results on a client assessment. Establishing goals includes identification of strategies for care and interventions and considers the need for resources. While the need for cost-effective care is always important, it should not be the primary focus of the case management plan. The plan should be multidisciplinary and should decrease the risk of negative outcomes.

118. B: A situation that requires termination of case management includes when the client has met the maximum allowable benefit for case management. The case manager should plan in advance for the termination, taking all possible steps to ensure the client's case management plan is adequate and can continue without direct supervision. Other reasons for termination include client wishes, achievement of goals, and a change in health care setting or type/level of care that precludes continued case management.

119. D: With a preferred provider organization, the client must always pay a deductible, which is a set amount that varies according to the plan but may range from $100 to $5,000 or more. Additionally, many plans now also require a copayment, which may be a percentage of the cost or (more commonly) a set amount, such as $25. With a PPO, clients are expected to see a physician from within a list of preferred providers. Some plans allow clients to seek care outside the PPO, but the clients' share of expenses increases.

120. B: Utilization Review Accreditation Commission (URAC) provides guidelines and staff training for case managers related to transitions of care, providing both case manager standards and performance measures. *Transitions of care* refer to changes the client encounters in locations, types and levels of care, and care providers. The program reviews the components of case management, methods for engaging customers in education, staff training, assessment and planning, coordination of care, and reporting. Measures include readmissions, worker's compensation, complaint responses, customer satisfaction, refusal of services transitions, and activation.

121. D: A warning sign that a case manager is developing a relationship with a client that is too personal is the case manager asking the client about personal matters unrelated to the client's needs. It's common to enjoy interacting with some clients more than others or even feel some attraction to a client, but the case manager should recognize signs and avoid acting on any attraction or showing preference for one client over others, while maintaining a professional relationship at all times.

122. A: When conducting an interview, the case manager should avoid questions that begin with "why" because they require the person being interviewed to provide a reason. Not only do some people find it difficult to explain their actions, but they also may simply feel providing reasons is an invasion of their privacy and intrusive. "Why" questions can also seem accusatory to some people, as if the case manager is finding fault with their actions or choices.

123. B: Under the Emergency Medical Treatment and Labor Act (EMTALA), emergency departments are legally required to provide a medical exam and stabilizing care to anyone who seeks care, regardless of the person's ability to pay. Once a client is stabilized, the client may be transferred to another facility, such as a county hospital that takes indigent clients. Various other services may be available to treat indigent clients, such as free clinics, and some hospitals, such as teaching hospitals, may provide free services.

124. A: When a client's condition does not progress according to expectations as outlined in the clinical pathway, this is referred to as a variance. For tracking purposes, when a variance occurs, it is classified according to where the cause lies—with the client, the physician, the nursing staff, other health care providers, or the system. A variance may result in a new pathway or an adjusted pathway, depending on the type of variance. In some cases, more than one pathway will be followed at the same time.

125. A: While these are four essential functions, the primary function of the case manager is coordination of care. The case manager collaborates with others in the health care team to provide day-to-day care and provide discharge planning as well as education for client and family. The case manager facilitates safe passage through the health care system and plans for appropriate follow-up clinical and community services. Consistent and effective coordination of care helps to promote cost-effective care as well by identifying problems and facilitating early intervention.

126. C: While all of these are important goals, the primary goal of community-based case management is to assist clients to access services in order to promote independent functioning. Community-based case managers must be familiar with health care and service providers in the community and should work closely with an interdisciplinary team, including social workers and appropriate therapists, in order to identify and attend to clients' needs. Clients and family members should be active participants in planning.

127. D: An appropriate statement for a case manager to make on a social networking site about working with clients is no statement whatsoever! The case manager should not describe clients, even in general terms without naming them, because people may be able to determine to whom the case manager refers by the description. Additionally, complaining about work ("I have to see way too many clients") suggests that the case manager is not able to give adequate attention to clients.

128. B: *Sentinel procedures* refers to those procedures (often diagnostic) associated with life-threatening diseases or conditions. When clients are undergoing sentinel procedures, this should alert the case manager for the potential need for case management services even if the initial diagnoses do not indicate a need, as the ultimate diagnosis may be far more life-threatening. Sentinel procedures includes exploratory laparotomy, organ (heart, lung, liver, kidney, brain, bone marrow) and lymph node biopsies, and insertion of arteriovenous shunt.

129. B: When doing financial analysis of diagnosis-related groups (DRGs), *relative weights* refers to value assigned to DRG based on complexity and resources needed. Complexity usually refers to the number of different services required for treatment. Some diagnoses may fall within only one DRG while other diagnoses may fall within a number of DRGs, all with different relative weights assigned. When relative weights are high, reimbursement increases, so some institutions may favor admissions with high relative weights.

130. C: A client who is temporarily disabled and has short-term disability insurance should usually expect to collect 60% of pre-disability salary after the client has used up all of the sick time. Short-term disability insurance usually covers a period of up to 6 months, although this may vary somewhat. However, clients must return to work when the disability is resolved, so many collect for only a brief period. Typical examples of short-term disabilities include pregnancy, back injuries, and fractures.

131. B: For consultation with a client and family to be effective, the case manager must first establish a trusting relationship. The case manager must begin by cultivating trust at the first visit by being honest, respecting the client's privacy, and persevering in order to establish credibility. The case manager should expect some resistance and testing but must remain nonjudgmental while clarifying the client's perception of issues and determining the effect the client's and family's beliefs, attitudes, and behaviors may have.

132. D: Domain is the term that refers to a case manager's area of practice and sphere of knowledge. Function comprises the actions that the case manager carries out in fulfilling the job requirements. Role refers to the function, job title, or position of the case manager. Venue (also referred to as context) refers to the specific type of organization or institution for which the case manager is employed and the type of population the case manager serves.

133. C: Motivational interviewing aims to help clients resolve their ambivalence about behavioral change. Change talk is an element of motivational interviewing and refers to statements that clients make indicating that they are committed to change. The interviewer's role is to help guide the client toward change talk, as there is a correlation between change talk and successful change in behavior. Change talk may proceed from statements about a desire and need to change to indications of a willingness to take steps to facilitate change.

134. D: A client who refuses to talk to the case manager because her husband had a bad experience with a case manager is exhibiting a barrier to communication involving perceptions. The client has a preconceived negative impression of the case manager and the case manager services based on her husband's experience, even though it may be totally unrelated. The case manager should acknowledge the problems the husband encountered and encourage the client to express her feelings openly to begin to build a relationship of trust.

135. C: Adherence to the plan of care is important if the goals of case management are to be met, but there may be many barriers to adherence (lack of income, need to work, lack of assistance, pain), so the best solution to lack of adherence is to sit down with the client and, in a nonjudgmental manner, discuss the client's goals and any barriers the client has encountered in order to determine what steps can be taken to improve adherence.

136. C: When doing telephonic case management, the primary focus is usually on triaging clients to determine which clients have emergent needs requiring immediate attention, urgent needs and can be referred to a primary care physician with 8 to 24 hours, and non-urgent needs and can provide self-care with guidance from the case manager. Case managers are commonly used in managed care organizations in order to prevent negative health outcomes and hospitalization, utilize resources wisely, and reduce costs.

137. C: If the case manager is concerned that a client's attention seems to wander, the best test to assess attention is the Digit Repetition Test. The client is asked to listen to numbers and then repeat them. The case manager starts with two random single-digit numbers. If the client gets this sequence correct, the case manager then states 3 numbers and continues to add one number each time until the client is unable to repeat the numbers correctly. People with normal intelligence (without retardation or expressive aphasia) can usually repeat 5 to 7 numbers, so scores < 5 indicate impaired attention.

138. B: The case manager may break a client's confidentiality only under limited circumstances, which include when a client is in need of emergent care and this care necessitates information (for example, if a client has taken an overdose of a particular drug). Other circumstances include when clients pose a risk of harm to themselves or others. Confidentiality may be breached when discussing the client's condition with a supervisor. Clients may be referred to collection services if they fail to pay for services in a reasonable time frame.

139. A: A bipolar client who is very nervous about transitioning into the community from a sheltered environment may benefit from a support group comprised of people dealing with similar issues. Support groups may have a mental health professional as a leader. Support groups are usually open groups that allow clients to choose whether or not to attend, but the groups provide a safe and supportive atmosphere where people can discuss shared concerns and methods of coping.

140. B: According to the American with Disabilities Act (ADA), public transportation must provide lifts that can accommodate occupied manual or powered wheelchairs that weigh up to 600 pounds. However, if the lift is able to support greater weight, the operator must accommodate those with weights greater than 600 pounds to the weight limit of the lift. The ADA also requires that the lifts accommodate wheelchairs up to 30 by 48 inches in width and length.

141. D: A client who insists that the case manager sit down with the client and explain the health care options in detail and outline them in writing is exhibiting self-advocacy by insisting on what he or she needs to understand and make decisions. Self-advocacy involves a client speaking up and becoming an active participant in planning and making decisions about care. Clients who advocate for themselves are more likely to want to be involved in self-care and to remain in compliance with treatment.

142. C: To increase compliance, the case manager who institutes changes in procedures in order to improve patient outcomes should include accountability. For example, a procedure may require that a checklist be completed and documented. Initially, the changes should be communicated and explained to staff, but this alone does not always bring about compliance because staff members often resort to familiar procedures, especially if they are busy and less familiar with the new procedure.

143. D: The primary purpose of predictive modeling is to identify clients at risk for negative outcomes because of their clinical condition, health history, and various other factors (pharmacy utilization, health insurance claims) so that the case manager can take a proactive approach to intervention and prevention. Predictive modeling produces a Risk Index (RI) that helps to identify clients who can benefit from case management. Predictive modeling may be used in conjunction with other forms of assessment, such as assessing client acuity.

144. A: Core indicators of end-stage disease are those that are common among a wide range of clients, regardless of diagnosis. Core indicators include serum albumin less than 2.5 g/dL, decline in physical condition, presence of multiple morbidities, assistance needed for most ADLs, Karnofsky score 50% or less, and the client expressing a desire to die. In addition to core indicators, there are disease-specific indicators. For example, stroke clients often exhibit decreased level of consciousness, dysphagia, dementia, and increased medical complications.

145. D: A hospice case manager is primarily responsible for coordinating services to provide care and comfort to the dying and their families. While pain management and emotional support are important elements of case management, and cost-effectiveness is always a concern, hospice clients often have multiple needs, which may include oxygen therapy, wound care, and nutritional support.

Caregivers may require respite or assistance, and families may have financial difficulties. The hospice case manager must view the client holistically in order to ensure that the client receives appropriate care and comfort.

146. C: The goal of a work hardening program is for the client to return to full work. Clients must usually be able to participate for at least 4 hours a day 3 to 5 days per week. Activities may include strengthening and mobility exercises; job practice or job simulation; training regarding safety issues, work pacing, work behaviors, and time management; and evaluation of the need for job modifications. Each client has an individualized plan with measurable goals and objectives.

147. D: If conducting a behavioral health assessment for a client who is noncompliant with treatment, the case manager should focus on the reason for the behavior rather the effects of how the behavior is exhibited. For example, the case manager should assess things such as the cost of treatment and the ability of the client to pay, the time needed for compliance activities and the other responsibilities the client has (children, work) that may interfere, and access to transportation.

148. A: Under Medicare A's inpatient prospective payment system, the organization should expect to be paid according to the payment classification of Medicare severity diagnosis-related group (MS-DRG). The MS-DRG is determined by the principal and secondary diagnoses (8 or less), ICD-10 procedures (6 or less), client's age, client's gender, and client's discharge status. Various other factors, including the hospital location and cost of living, are used to calculate the hospital-specific prices. Hospitals serving large numbers of low-income clients and teaching hospitals may receive additional payment.

149. C: While all of these are important considerations for the client with multiple comorbidities and multiple physicians, these clients are especially at risk for polypharmacy so one of the first assessments should be medication reconciliation. This should be done initially and after any intervention, such as a visit to the physician or a hospitalization. The case manager should assess the medications, the prescribing physicians, the client's knowledge about the medications, and the client's method, dosage, and frequency of taking the medications; clients often fail to take medications as prescribed.

150. D: Clients with schizophrenia, depression, or bipolar disease are at high risk for dual diagnosis as many clients self-medicate with alcohol or illicit drugs. These clients often need enrollment in a program that targets both problems, as the approach to treatment for substance abuse is different for mentally ill clients than for those who are not mentally ill. Programs for dual diagnosis clients tend to be more supportive and less confrontational. Peer support is also important to treatment.

151. B: The case manager should always avoid dual relationships with clients. While it is unethical to have a sexual or romantic relationship with a client, serious problems can also arise if the case manager has other relationships with a client. The case manager should not work with neighbors, friends, relatives, or other acquaintances because the case manager is in the position of power, making decisions about the client's care; this may result in perceptions of abuse of power or conflict of interest.

152. D: Self-directed Medicaid services allow participants to make decisions over certain specified services. The participant may use Medicaid funds to hire a personal aide or an individual person to provide care that would otherwise be done by the client or a skilled provider. For example, a client no longer able to do intermittent catheterization may be allowed to hire, train, and supervise an individual person or personal aide to do this procedure. Self-directed Medicaid services may include both "employer authority" (hiring, training, supervising) and "budget authority" (determining how funds are distributed).

153. D: Utilization management is done to determine if the use of services, facilities, and procedures is appropriate and medically necessary. Utilization management requires analysis of:

- Misutilization: Treatment errors or other inefficient processes, such as scheduling problems
- Overutilization: Inappropriate admissions, inappropriate length of stay, inappropriate levels of care, and inadequate documentation for use of resources (such as diagnostic testing)
- Underutilization: Failure to admit, inadequate diagnostic testing, inadequate levels of care
- Interventions should be planned based on the outcomes of this analysis, considering cost-effectiveness and process improvement strategies

154. B: When documenting a verbal exchange with a client, the case manager must avoid subjective opinions and provide an objective report: "Client states treatment is not working and, therefore, refused to take medications." Whenever possible, the reason for the client's action should be included, not just that the client is refusing treatment, because the information that the client believes the treatment is ineffective is important for healthcare workers to address with the client.

155. A: The case manager realizes that when a client transitions between providers, the client is at increased risk for complication and negative outcomes because the new provider (whether in a different level of care or in a different facility) may have insufficient knowledge of the client's condition and history. Inadequate communication may result in incorrect treatments, medication errors, and neglect of client needs. New providers may not be clear about who is responsible for different aspects of care, so the case manager must ensure continuity of care.

156. C: For a client covered by Medicare A for rehabilitation hospitalization, the admission FIM scores must be obtained during the first 3 calendar days, and the scores should be based on activities the client performs during the entire 3 days. A 3-day discharge assessment window is also used for the discharge FIM score, but the assessment must be completed within any 24-hour period within those 3 days (except for assessment of bowel and bladder function, which requires 3 days for assistance and 7 days for incontinence).

157. D: The Rancho Los Amigos Levels of Cognitive Functioning tool is used to evaluate traumatic brain injuries. According to the tool, a client with a score of VIII is exhibiting appropriate behavior. The scale runs from I to VIII with I at one end of the scale indicating unresponsiveness to all types of stimuli and VIII at the other end of the scale (purposeful, appropriate response). A revised scale (I to X) is also used in some places and includes descriptions of ability to function (needs assistance, independent).

158. A: The primary goal of quality improvement projects is to evaluate where and how medical errors occur rather than to assign blame. Reducing errors often serves to increase cost savings. Errors may include failure to provide adequate care and inefficient procedures, as well as direct errors, such as giving the wrong medication. Objectives include reducing the overall medical errors and associated morbidities and mortality, developing best practices, improving client satisfaction with care, promoting safety, and improving professional performance of duties.

159. D: If an uninsured client who is ineligible for Medicaid is unable to pay for an expensive chemotherapeutic drug, the initial step in solving the problem is to determine if the drug company has a pharmaceutical assistance program. Most drug companies have such programs, usually intended for those who are uninsured or underinsured and meet specific criteria for need. Some programs are drug-specific. Some states also have pharmaceutical assistance programs, especially for AIDS drugs.

160. A: Generally, the most important factor in whether a purchaser profits from a viatical settlement is the length of time the insured lives after purchase. The purchaser of another's life insurance plan generally tries to pay as far below face value as possible because plans usually require continued monthly payments. Viatical settlements are generally profitable if the covered person dies within 2 years, but if the person lives for 10 to 20 years, then the purchaser may lose money.

161. C: In order to meet the "recent work test" for SSDI, a client who becomes disabled in the quarter when he turns 30 years old must have worked half of the years since the quarter after turning 21, or 4.5 years out of the 9 years that have elapsed. Those who become disabled on or before the quarter of turning 24 must have worked 1.5 years out of the preceding 3 years, and those 31 or older must have worked at least 5 out of the preceding 10 years.

162. A: When conducting a client needs assessment as part of caseload calculations, the most important factors are:

- Acuity: Includes clinical characteristics. Increased clinical needs, such as with multiple morbidities or severe trauma, increased need for case manager time.
- Personal and family psychosocial issues: Issues may include cognitive impairment, psychological or mental illness, conflict, spiritual needs, ability of family/caregivers to assist in client care, needs of family and caregivers, and belief systems.
- Environment: Includes transitions of care.

163. B: With the accelerated rapid-cycle change approach to quality improvement, the team members focus on identifying solutions rather than analysis. There are 4 areas of concern in this method:

- Models for rapid-cycle change: Doubling or tripling the rate of quality improvement by modifying and accelerating traditional methods
- Pre-work: Problem statements, graphic demonstrations of data, flowcharts, and literature review. Team members identified
- Team creation: Rapid action (also sometimes rapid acceleration or rapid achievement) teams (RATs) formed
- Team meetings and workflow: Meetings/work scheduled over 6 weeks from initial work to implementation

164. D: Health insurance is based on the principle of risk pooling. The insurance company enrolls large numbers of applicants, assuming that not all applicants will require payouts, so that the company can pay out benefits to only a portion of the applicants and still make a substantial profit. The law of large numbers is utilized to determine statistical probabilities related to mortality and morbidity in a specific time frame based on the pool of applicants.

165. D: CHAMPVA requires preauthorization for hospice services, durable medical equipment with cost of purchase or rental of $2,000 or more, mental health services, substance abuse service, transplants (organ/bone marrow), and dental procedures associated with medical conditions. Diagnostic procedures and referrals to specialists do not require preauthorization if they are medically necessary. CHAMPVA provides health care coverage for spouses and children of disabled veterans or veterans who died in the line of duty. Those eligible for TRICARE are not also eligible for CHAMPVA.

166. A: Storming. Tuckman's stages of group development:

- Forming: Leader takes active role and members follow.
- Storming: Opinions diverge and conflict may occur. Resistance may occur as shown by the absence of members, shared silence, and subgroup formation.
- Norming: Members begin to express positive feelings toward each other and feel attached to the group.
- Performing: Leader's input and direction decreases and focuses primarily on keeping the members on track with tasks.
- Mourning: The group disbands or leader/members leave the group.

167. B: If a client with a disability is applying for a job and asks the case manager if he should disclose the disability to the employer, the best response is, "You only need to disclose if you expect an accommodation." If no accommodation is needed for the client to carry out job functions, then there is no legal requirement under the American with Disabilities Act for the client to disclose the information, and it is not legal for the employer to ask if an applicant has a disability. However, if informed about the disability, the employer can ask what accommodations, if any, are needed.

168. D: Resource utilization groups (RUGs) and minimum data sets (MDSs) are used to establish payment rates for skilled nursing facilities and help determine reimbursement under Medicare's PPS program. There are currently 53 RUGs with the RUG determined by the client's ADL score, use of therapy (based on minutes of therapy), services (intravenous therapy, respiratory therapy), functional ability, and medical conditions. The MDS is an assessment instrument used to evaluate service use and client characteristics.

169. A: If the case manager is utilizing video calls with clients rather than in-person visits, the HIPAA regulations regarding privacy and security must apply. Therefore, the video calls must be encrypted so that the calls cannot be accessed by others. The Privacy Rule protects any information in the medical record, billing information, conversations between the client and case manager, and other health information. The security rule requires that electronic health information be secure and protected and safeguards be in place.

170. B: According to the Transtheoretical Model of change, the process of change that people go through when they express feelings (positive and negative) about change is dramatic relief. People go through 5 stages when attempting to change: precontemplation, contemplation, preparation, action, and maintenance. People also go through 10 processes at each stage of change. Processes include consciousness raising, counterconditioning, dramatic relief, environmental reevaluation, helping relationships, reinforcement management, self-liberation, self-evaluation, social liberation, and stimulus control.

171. A: In order to qualify for inpatient rehabilitation, a client must be able to undergo rehabilitation therapy for at least 3 hours daily for 5 to 7 days per week. If clients require therapy but cannot tolerate this many hours of therapy, then they may be transferred to a skilled nursing facility, which requires that the clients need skilled care daily (including rehabilitation therapy and/or medical treatments) and are medically stable. Sub-acute care is available for clients who do not still require acute care but require more care than is available in a skilled nursing facility.

172. C: An example of an appropriate documentation for a client who appears inebriated during a face-to-face visit is "Client unsteady on feet, speech is slurred, and smells of alcohol." Subjective statements and assumptions, such as "appeared inebriated" and "from drinking" must be avoided. Statements must be objective and as observed. Avoiding the situation by documenting that the "client needed to reschedule visit" is not a factual representation.

173. D: In the Patient-Centered Medical Home Model of care, the team leader coordinating care is usually the client's personal physician with whom the client has an ongoing relationship; the physician understands the needs of the client and can lead the team in providing the resources the client needs throughout the patient's life stages and continuum of care. The physician serves as a patient advocate and utilizes evidence-based practices and clinical decision support tools and information technology as well as continuous quality improvement. Clients are active participants in care.

174. A: While all of these strategies are used to contain pharmaceutical costs, the most common strategy is the use of generic drugs rather than brand-name drugs. This strategy alone may save up to 80% of the cost of drugs, depending on the medications and the volume. Pharmacy benefit programs often require a substantially larger copay for non-generic drugs or require the person to pay the entire cost. Prescription forms usually contain a place where physicians can agree to generic substitutions.

175. D: The most important factor in cost management is eliminating duplication of services and care fragmentation. The case manager may also manage costs by conducting cost comparisons when obtaining supplies and equipment, but the least expensive option is not always the best, so quality is also a consideration. The case manager may exercise creativity and ingenuity in providing services in a cost-effective manner. The case manager may need to actively obtain data in order to show cost-effectiveness and influence coverage by the individual's insurance carrier.

176. A: Failure to rescue (FTR) is a term used in reporting mortality rates and refers specifically to the inability to identify life-threatening complications in time to prevent death through appropriate interventions. Overall FTR rates have decreased because of fewer postoperative complications, but FTR rates have increased in some areas, such as urologic procedures. Clients at increased risk of FTR include the elderly, clients with severe illness, ethnic minorities, Medicaid clients, and clients at urban hospitals.

177. B: The Chronic Care Model is primarily utilized in the primary care setting and focuses on providing case management to those with chronic illnesses in order to improve client outcomes through prevention. Clients are considered active participants in their own care. The components of the model include the health system that is involved, the delivery system of care (team members and roles), the use of evidence-based guidelines for decision support and integrated care of primary physician and specialists, clinical information systems, and utilization of community resources.

178. B: The purpose of the Patient Activation Measure (PAM) is to assess the client's ability for self-care by evaluating knowledge about medications and condition and confidence in managing care. This instrument assesses 13 items with scores ranging from 0 (low ability) to 52 (high ability). Clients are placed into one of four levels of self-care based on their scores:

- Level 1: Client's role is passive.
- Level 2: Client lacks confidence in abilities and adequate understanding of health.
- Level 3: Client is beginning to build understanding, but still may lack confidence.
- Level 4: Client is managing self-care, but may falter with stress or health problems.

179. C: A case manager who influences members of a group but is not in turn influenced by the members is exemplifying unilateral interdependence. Interdependence occurs when people's attitudes, experiences, and feelings are influenced by someone else. With unilateral interdependence, the leader influences the followers but the lack of mutual influence suggests an autocratic relationship, which may be useful in emergent situations but may impair group dynamics as followers feel they have no voice.

180. C: In order to qualify for SSI, the maximum limit for resources for a married couple is $3,000. Resources include cash, savings accounts, stocks and bonds, land, vehicles, personal property, life insurance, and anything else of significant value that be sold. Those who are eligible include those 65 years and older and those who are blind or disabled with limited income and resources. Applicants must be US citizens or within an eligible category of aliens (such as Amerasians and Cubans).

CCM Practice Test #3

To take this additional CCM practice test, visit our bonus page:
mometrix.com/bonus948/ccm

How to Overcome Test Anxiety

Just the thought of taking a test is enough to make most people a little nervous. A test is an important event that can have a long-term impact on your future, so it's important to take it seriously and it's natural to feel anxious about performing well. But just because anxiety is normal, that doesn't mean that it's helpful in test taking, or that you should simply accept it as part of your life. Anxiety can have a variety of effects. These effects can be mild, like making you feel slightly nervous, or severe, like blocking your ability to focus or remember even a simple detail.

If you experience test anxiety—whether severe or mild—it's important to know how to beat it. To discover this, first you need to understand what causes test anxiety.

Causes of Test Anxiety

While we often think of anxiety as an uncontrollable emotional state, it can actually be caused by simple, practical things. One of the most common causes of test anxiety is that a person does not feel adequately prepared for their test. This feeling can be the result of many different issues such as poor study habits or lack of organization, but the most common culprit is time management. Starting to study too late, failing to organize your study time to cover all of the material, or being distracted while you study will mean that you're not well prepared for the test. This may lead to cramming the night before, which will cause you to be physically and mentally exhausted for the test. Poor time management also contributes to feelings of stress, fear, and hopelessness as you realize you are not well prepared but don't know what to do about it.

Other times, test anxiety is not related to your preparation for the test but comes from unresolved fear. This may be a past failure on a test, or poor performance on tests in general. It may come from comparing yourself to others who seem to be performing better or from the stress of living up to expectations. Anxiety may be driven by fears of the future—how failure on this test would affect your educational and career goals. These fears are often completely irrational, but they can still negatively impact your test performance.

Elements of Test Anxiety

As mentioned earlier, test anxiety is considered to be an emotional state, but it has physical and mental components as well. Sometimes you may not even realize that you are suffering from test anxiety until you notice the physical symptoms. These can include trembling hands, rapid heartbeat, sweating, nausea, and tense muscles. Extreme anxiety may lead to fainting or vomiting. Obviously, any of these symptoms can have a negative impact on testing. It is important to recognize them as soon as they begin to occur so that you can address the problem before it damages your performance.

The mental components of test anxiety include trouble focusing and inability to remember learned information. During a test, your mind is on high alert, which can help you recall information and stay focused for an extended period of time. However, anxiety interferes with your mind's natural processes, causing you to blank out, even on the questions you know well. The strain of testing during anxiety makes it difficult to stay focused, especially on a test that may take several hours. Extreme anxiety can take a huge mental toll, making it difficult not only to recall test information but even to understand the test questions or pull your thoughts together.

Effects of Test Anxiety

Test anxiety is like a disease—if left untreated, it will get progressively worse. Anxiety leads to poor performance, and this reinforces the feelings of fear and failure, which in turn lead to poor performances on subsequent tests. It can grow from a mild nervousness to a crippling condition. If allowed to progress, test anxiety can have a big impact on your schooling, and consequently on your future.

Test anxiety can spread to other parts of your life. Anxiety on tests can become anxiety in any stressful situation, and blanking on a test can turn into panicking in a job situation. But fortunately, you don't have to let anxiety rule your testing and determine your grades. There are a number of relatively simple steps you can take to move past anxiety and function normally on a test and in the rest of life.

Physical Steps for Beating Test Anxiety

While test anxiety is a serious problem, the good news is that it can be overcome. It doesn't have to control your ability to think and remember information. While it may take time, you can begin taking steps today to beat anxiety.

Just as your first hint that you may be struggling with anxiety comes from the physical symptoms, the first step to treating it is also physical. Rest is crucial for having a clear, strong mind. If you are tired, it is much easier to give in to anxiety. But if you establish good sleep habits, your body and mind will be ready to perform optimally, without the strain of exhaustion. Additionally, sleeping well helps you to retain information better, so you're more likely to recall the answers when you see the test questions.

Getting good sleep means more than going to bed on time. It's important to allow your brain time to relax. Take study breaks from time to time so it doesn't get overworked, and don't study right before bed. Take time to rest your mind before trying to rest your body, or you may find it difficult to fall asleep.

Along with sleep, other aspects of physical health are important in preparing for a test. Good nutrition is vital for good brain function. Sugary foods and drinks may give a burst of energy but this burst is followed by a crash, both physically and emotionally. Instead, fuel your body with protein and vitamin-rich foods.

Also, drink plenty of water. Dehydration can lead to headaches and exhaustion, especially if your brain is already under stress from the rigors of the test. Particularly if your test is a long one, drink water during the breaks. And if possible, take an energy-boosting snack to eat between sections.

Along with sleep and diet, a third important part of physical health is exercise. Maintaining a steady workout schedule is helpful, but even taking 5-minute study breaks to walk can help get your blood pumping faster and clear your head. Exercise also releases endorphins, which contribute to a positive feeling and can help combat test anxiety.

When you nurture your physical health, you are also contributing to your mental health. If your body is healthy, your mind is much more likely to be healthy as well. So take time to rest, nourish your body with healthy food and water, and get moving as much as possible. Taking these physical steps will make you stronger and more able to take the mental steps necessary to overcome test anxiety.

Mental Steps for Beating Test Anxiety

Working on the mental side of test anxiety can be more challenging, but as with the physical side, there are clear steps you can take to overcome it. As mentioned earlier, test anxiety often stems from lack of preparation, so the obvious solution is to prepare for the test. Effective studying may be the most important weapon you have for beating test anxiety, but you can and should employ several other mental tools to combat fear.

First, boost your confidence by reminding yourself of past success—tests or projects that you aced. If you're putting as much effort into preparing for this test as you did for those, there's no reason you should expect to fail here. Work hard to prepare; then trust your preparation.

Second, surround yourself with encouraging people. It can be helpful to find a study group, but be sure that the people you're around will encourage a positive attitude. If you spend time with others who are anxious or cynical, this will only contribute to your own anxiety. Look for others who are motivated to study hard from a desire to succeed, not from a fear of failure.

Third, reward yourself. A test is physically and mentally tiring, even without anxiety, and it can be helpful to have something to look forward to. Plan an activity following the test, regardless of the outcome, such as going to a movie or getting ice cream.

When you are taking the test, if you find yourself beginning to feel anxious, remind yourself that you know the material. Visualize successfully completing the test. Then take a few deep, relaxing breaths and return to it. Work through the questions carefully but with confidence, knowing that you are capable of succeeding.

Developing a healthy mental approach to test taking will also aid in other areas of life. Test anxiety affects more than just the actual test—it can be damaging to your mental health and even contribute to depression. It's important to beat test anxiety before it becomes a problem for more than testing.

Study Strategy

Being prepared for the test is necessary to combat anxiety, but what does being prepared look like? You may study for hours on end and still not feel prepared. What you need is a strategy for test prep. The next few pages outline our recommended steps to help you plan out and conquer the challenge of preparation.

Step 1: Scope Out the Test

Learn everything you can about the format (multiple choice, essay, etc.) and what will be on the test. Gather any study materials, course outlines, or sample exams that may be available. Not only will this help you to prepare, but knowing what to expect can help to alleviate test anxiety.

Step 2: Map Out the Material

Look through the textbook or study guide and make note of how many chapters or sections it has. Then divide these over the time you have. For example, if a book has 15 chapters and you have five days to study, you need to cover three chapters each day. Even better, if you have the time, leave an extra day at the end for overall review after you have gone through the material in depth.

If time is limited, you may need to prioritize the material. Look through it and make note of which sections you think you already have a good grasp on, and which need review. While you are studying, skim quickly through the familiar sections and take more time on the challenging parts.

Write out your plan so you don't get lost as you go. Having a written plan also helps you feel more in control of the study, so anxiety is less likely to arise from feeling overwhelmed at the amount to cover.

Step 3: Gather Your Tools

Decide what study method works best for you. Do you prefer to highlight in the book as you study and then go back over the highlighted portions? Or do you type out notes of the important information? Or is it helpful to make flashcards that you can carry with you? Assemble the pens, index cards, highlighters, post-it notes, and any other materials you may need so you won't be distracted by getting up to find things while you study.

If you're having a hard time retaining the information or organizing your notes, experiment with different methods. For example, try color-coding by subject with colored pens, highlighters, or post-it notes. If you learn better by hearing, try recording yourself reading your notes so you can listen while in the car, working out, or simply sitting at your desk. Ask a friend to quiz you from your flashcards, or try teaching someone the material to solidify it in your mind.

Step 4: Create Your Environment

It's important to avoid distractions while you study. This includes both the obvious distractions like visitors and the subtle distractions like an uncomfortable chair (or a too-comfortable couch that makes you want to fall asleep). Set up the best study environment possible: good lighting and a comfortable work area. If background music helps you focus, you may want to turn it on, but otherwise keep the room quiet. If you are using a computer to take notes, be sure you don't have any other windows open, especially applications like social media, games, or anything else that could distract you. Silence your phone and turn off notifications. Be sure to keep water close by so you stay hydrated while you study (but avoid unhealthy drinks and snacks).

Also, take into account the best time of day to study. Are you freshest first thing in the morning? Try to set aside some time then to work through the material. Is your mind clearer in the afternoon or evening? Schedule your study session then. Another method is to study at the same time of day that you will take the test, so that your brain gets used to working on the material at that time and will be ready to focus at test time.

Step 5: Study!

Once you have done all the study preparation, it's time to settle into the actual studying. Sit down, take a few moments to settle your mind so you can focus, and begin to follow your study plan. Don't give in to distractions or let yourself procrastinate. This is your time to prepare so you'll be ready to fearlessly approach the test. Make the most of the time and stay focused.

Of course, you don't want to burn out. If you study too long you may find that you're not retaining the information very well. Take regular study breaks. For example, taking five minutes out of every hour to walk briskly, breathing deeply and swinging your arms, can help your mind stay fresh.

As you get to the end of each chapter or section, it's a good idea to do a quick review. Remind yourself of what you learned and work on any difficult parts. When you feel that you've mastered the material, move on to the next part. At the end of your study session, briefly skim through your notes again.

But while review is helpful, cramming last minute is NOT. If at all possible, work ahead so that you won't need to fit all your study into the last day. Cramming overloads your brain with more information than it can process and retain, and your tired mind may struggle to recall even previously learned information when it is overwhelmed with last-minute study. Also, the urgent nature of cramming and the stress placed on your brain contribute to anxiety. You'll be more likely to go to the test feeling unprepared and having trouble thinking clearly.

So don't cram, and don't stay up late before the test, even just to review your notes at a leisurely pace. Your brain needs rest more than it needs to go over the information again. In fact, plan to finish your studies by noon or early afternoon the day before the test. Give your brain the rest of the day to relax or focus on other things, and get a good night's sleep. Then you will be fresh for the test and better able to recall what you've studied.

Step 6: Take a Practice Test

Many courses offer sample tests, either online or in the study materials. This is an excellent resource to check whether you have mastered the material, as well as to prepare for the test format and environment.

Check the test format ahead of time: the number of questions, the type (multiple choice, free response, etc.), and the time limit. Then create a plan for working through them. For example, if you have 30 minutes to take a 60-question test, your limit is 30 seconds per question. Spend less time on the questions you know well so that you can take more time on the difficult ones.

If you have time to take several practice tests, take the first one open book, with no time limit. Work through the questions at your own pace and make sure you fully understand them. Gradually work up to taking a test under test conditions: sit at a desk with all study materials put away and set a timer. Pace yourself to make sure you finish the test with time to spare and go back to check your answers if you have time.

After each test, check your answers. On the questions you missed, be sure you understand why you missed them. Did you misread the question (tests can use tricky wording)? Did you forget the information? Or was it something you hadn't learned? Go back and study any shaky areas that the practice tests reveal.

Taking these tests not only helps with your grade, but also aids in combating test anxiety. If you're already used to the test conditions, you're less likely to worry about it, and working through tests until you're scoring well gives you a confidence boost. Go through the practice tests until you feel comfortable, and then you can go into the test knowing that you're ready for it.

Test Tips

On test day, you should be confident, knowing that you've prepared well and are ready to answer the questions. But aside from preparation, there are several test day strategies you can employ to maximize your performance.

First, as stated before, get a good night's sleep the night before the test (and for several nights before that, if possible). Go into the test with a fresh, alert mind rather than staying up late to study.

Try not to change too much about your normal routine on the day of the test. It's important to eat a nutritious breakfast, but if you normally don't eat breakfast at all, consider eating just a protein bar. If you're a coffee drinker, go ahead and have your normal coffee. Just make sure you time it so that the caffeine doesn't wear off right in the middle of your test. Avoid sugary beverages, and drink enough water to stay hydrated but not so much that you need a restroom break 10 minutes into the test. If your test isn't first thing in the morning, consider going for a walk or doing a light workout before the test to get your blood flowing.

Allow yourself enough time to get ready, and leave for the test with plenty of time to spare so you won't have the anxiety of scrambling to arrive in time. Another reason to be early is to select a good seat. It's helpful to sit away from doors and windows, which can be distracting. Find a good seat, get out your supplies, and settle your mind before the test begins.

When the test begins, start by going over the instructions carefully, even if you already know what to expect. Make sure you avoid any careless mistakes by following the directions.

Then begin working through the questions, pacing yourself as you've practiced. If you're not sure on an answer, don't spend too much time on it, and don't let it shake your confidence. Either skip it and come back later, or eliminate as many wrong answers as possible and guess among the remaining ones. Don't dwell on these questions as you continue—put them out of your mind and focus on what lies ahead.

Be sure to read all of the answer choices, even if you're sure the first one is the right answer. Sometimes you'll find a better one if you keep reading. But don't second-guess yourself if you do immediately know the answer. Your gut instinct is usually right. Don't let test anxiety rob you of the information you know.

If you have time at the end of the test (and if the test format allows), go back and review your answers. Be cautious about changing any, since your first instinct tends to be correct, but make sure you didn't misread any of the questions or accidentally mark the wrong answer choice. Look over any you skipped and make an educated guess.

At the end, leave the test feeling confident. You've done your best, so don't waste time worrying about your performance or wishing you could change anything. Instead, celebrate the successful completion of this test. And finally, use this test to learn how to deal with anxiety even better next time.

Review Video: Test Anxiety
Visit mometrix.com/academy and enter code: 100340

Important Qualification

Not all anxiety is created equal. If your test anxiety is causing major issues in your life beyond the classroom or testing center, or if you are experiencing troubling physical symptoms related to your anxiety, it may be a sign of a serious physiological or psychological condition. If this sounds like your situation, we strongly encourage you to seek professional help.

Additional Bonus Material

Due to our efforts to try to keep this book to a manageable length, we've created a link that will give you access to all of your additional bonus material:

mometrix.com/bonus948/ccm

www.ingramcontent.com/pod-product-compliance
Lightning Source LLC
Chambersburg PA
CBHW061404210326
41598CB00035B/6090